I0128103

William Gilbert Anderson

Light Gymnastics

A Guide to Systematic Instruction in Physical Training

William Gilbert Anderson

Light Gymnastics
A Guide to Systematic Instruction in Physical Training

ISBN/EAN: 9783337251253

Printed in Europe, USA, Canada, Australia, Japan

Cover: Foto ©Paul-Georg Meister /pixelio.de

More available books at **www.hansebooks.com**

LIGHT GYMNASTICS.

A GUIDE

TO

SYSTEMATIC INSTRUCTION IN PHYSICAL TRAINING.

FOR USE IN SCHOOLS, GYMNASIA, ETC.

BY

WILLIAM G. ANDERSON, M.D., F.SS.,

*President of the Brooklyn Normal School for Physical Education; Physician in
charge of the Department of Physical Education, Adelphi Academy, Brooklyn,
N. Y.; Director of the Department of Physical Education, Chautauqua
University, Chautauqua, N. Y.; Secretary of the American
Association for the Advancement of Physical Education;
Member of Victoria Institute, London; Director of
Physical Education, Long Island College
Hospital, etc. etc.*

Fully Illustrated.

NEW YORK:

EFFINGHAM MAYNARD & CO., PUBLISHERS,

771 BROADWAY AND 67 & 69 NINTH ST.

1890.

THIS SIMPLE VOLUME

IS AFFECTIONATELY INSCRIBED TO

My Wife,

TO WHOM I AM INDEBTED MORE THAN TO ALL OTHERS

FOR READY AID AND ASSISTANCE.

Copyright, 1889, by Effingham Maynard & Co.

PREFACE.

IT is now generally admitted by educators that the pupils in our institutions of learning need some kind of systematized physical training in connection with their mental work.

The action of the foremost educators in the world, the faculties of our leading colleges, permitting the expenditure of many hundreds of thousands of dollars on magnificent gymnasiums, strengthens the assertion. The example thus set must be and is being followed by the public and private schools. They are gradually introducing gymnastics as a part of their course of study.

Teachers are responsible for the physical condition of their pupils while in their charge. If they are ignorant of the simple laws of health and gymnastics, their pupils will suffer on account of it.

It may be said in the teachers' defense, however, that should they desire the knowledge that would fit them to teach physical training from professional teachers of the subject, they could spare neither the time nor money to acquire it; consequently they must obtain this from books.

A good work on light gymnastics should be the

result of years of experience of a teacher of this subject. It should be compiled after a definite plan, be profusely illustrated, and contain exercises that are at the same time beneficial, simple, and of pleasing variety. In short, it should be a book that will be valuable to any teacher, because it is founded on fact and not fancy, and its methods such that any intelligent teacher can make use of them with success in his classes.

This has been the author's aim in making this manual. The subjects are treated from the standpoint of a physician and gymnastic director. The experience of years as an instructor of many thousands of pupils and teachers, the writer has endeavored to condense and simplify, in hopes that it may be of use to others.

He wishes to thank Dr. A. C. Perkins of the Adelphi Academy for the suggestions he has so kindly given; Mr. Henry S. Anderson for his assistance and aid; and Mr. Julius A. Pfarre for the use of cuts.

The drawings for military methods were made by L. J. Pennock of the Brooklyn Normal School for Physical Education.

MARCHING OR MILITARY METHODS.

File.—A row of scholars ranged one behind the other from front to rear.

Line or Rank.—A row of scholars placed side by side.

Guide.—The one who directs or leads a line of four or more.

Dress.—To straighten.

By right or left flank.—The same as a right or left face, but applicable only to scholars when marching.

Align.—To arrange according to height.

Pivot.—The one who makes the shortest turn in a wheel.

COMMANDS.

There are two kinds :

The *preparatory command*, such as *Forward*, which indicates the movement that is to be executed.

The command of *execution*, such as MARCH! or HALT!, the part of the command which causes the execution.

The preparatory commands are distinguished by *italics*, those of execution by SMALL CAPITALS.

The tone of command should be animated and distinct.

The instructor should never require a movement to be made until he has fully explained and executed it. He accustoms a pupil to take by himself the proper position, rectifies it when necessary, and sees that no movements are performed carelessly or with undue haste. Each movement should be understood before passing to another. After they have been properly executed in the order laid down, the instructor no longer confines himself to that order ; on the contrary, changes it to suit his wishes.

A MANUAL OF PHYSICAL TRAINING.

CHAPTER I.

THE POSITION OF ATTENTION.

HEELS on the same line and as near each other as the conformation of the body permits.

Feet turned out at an angle formed by the foot-marks (60°).

Knees straight.

The body erect on the hips, inclining a little forward.

Shoulders square and falling equally.

Elbows near the body.

Palms of the hands turned slightly to the front, arms hanging naturally.

The head erect. Chin slightly drawn in without constraint. Eyes to the front.

TO REST AND DISMISS SCHOLARS.

The teacher lets the pupils rest from time to time. For this purpose he commands, (1) *Squad*, (2) REST! At the command *rest*, the pupil is no longer required to preserve immobility, silence, or to remain strictly in his place.

If the instructor commands, (1) *In place*, (2) REST!,

7

the pupil is not required to preserve immobility or to keep strict silence, but must always keep one of his heels in place.

To resume attention the instructor commands, (1) *Company*, (2) ATTENTION! At the second command the pupil takes his position and remains motionless.

To dismiss the class the instructor commands, (1) *Break ranks*, (2) MARCH!

FACINGS.

To the Right or Left.—Command, (1) *Right*, or *Left*, (2) FACE! At the command *face*, raise the right foot slightly, face to the right, turning on the left heel, the left toe slightly raised ; replace the right heel by the side of the left and on the same line. The facings to the left are executed upon the same heel as the facings to the right.

To the Rear.—Command, (1) *Squad*, (2) ABOUT, (3) FACE! At the command *about*, turn on the left heel, bring the left toe to the front, carry the right foot to the rear, the hollow opposite to and three inches from the left heel, the feet square to each other. At the command *face*, turn on both heels, raise the toes a little, face to the rear, and when the face is nearly completed raise the right foot and replace it by the side of the left.

The German method of about facing is simple and saves time. It is executed after the manner of a right face, but the pupil turns half-way round instead of one quarter of a circle.

TO MARK TIME.

Being in march, the instructor commands, (1) *Mark time*, (2) MARK! At the second command, given the instant one foot is coming to the ground, continue the cadence and make a semblance of marching without gaining ground by alternately advancing each foot about half its length and bringing it back on a line with the other.

To resume the direct step command, (1) *Forward*, (2) MARCH

TO MARCH IN A DIRECT LINE.

Command, (1) *Forward*, (2) MARCH! At the command *march* advance the left foot about twenty inches from heel to heel, plant it, and in a like manner advance the right. Keep this movement up, the instructor indicating from time to time the cadence by calling *one, two, three, four*, or *left, right*.

To arrest the march the instructor commands, (1) *Company*, (2) HALT! At the command *halt*, given the instant either foot is brought to the ground, the foot in the rear is brought up and planted by the other.

A simple method of marking time is to permit the scholar to stamp the left foot lightly on the first of each four counts. It teaches children to catch the step quickly. This method has been used in running.

CADENCE.

For the purpose of this manual the following will be cadence or time :

Common time, 64 to 70 steps in one minute.

Quick time, 110 steps in one minute.

Double time, 190 steps in one minute.

SHORT STEP.

Being in the march the instructor commands, (1) *Short step*, (2) MARCH! At the second command the length of the step is reduced to 10 inches, the class resuming full step at the command, (1) *Forward*, (2) MARCH!

TO CHANGE STEP.

Being in march the instructor commands, (1) *Change step*, (2) MARCH! At the command *march*, given the instant the right foot comes to the ground, the left foot is advanced and planted; the hollow of the right foot is then advanced against the heel of the left, the pupil again stepping off with the left.

The change on the right foot is similarly executed, the command *march* being given when the left foot strikes the ground.

SIDE STEP.

Being at a halt, the instructor commands, (1) *Side step to the right*, or *left*, (2) MARCH! At the command *march*, carry the right foot six inches to the right, keeping the knees straight and the shoulders square to the front; as soon as the right foot is planted bring the left foot to the side of it and continue the movement, observing the cadence, until the commands, (1) *Squad*, (2) HALT!

In class work the side step is always executed in common time, unless quick time is specified.

BACK STEP.

Being at a halt, the instructor commands, (1) *Backward*, (2) MARCH! At the command *march*, step off smartly with the left foot fourteen inches straight to the rear, measuring from heel to heel, and so on with the feet in succession till the commands, (1) *Company*, (2) HALT!

At the command *halt* bring back the foot in front to the side of the one in rear.

TO MARCH TO THE REAR.

Being in march, the instructor commands, (1) *To the rear*, (2) MARCH! At the command *march*, given as the right foot strikes the ground, advance and plant the left foot; then turn on the balls of both feet, face to the right about, and immediately step off with the left foot.

DOUBLE TIME.

The instructor commands, (1) *Forward, double time*, (2) MARCH! At the first command raise the hands till the fore-arms are horizontal, fingers closed, nails toward body, elbows to the rear. At next command, quicken the step until all are in a slow run (190 steps a minute), when the instructor will indicate the cadence by counting one, two, given alternately, as the left and right foot touch the ground.

To come to slow time the instructor commands, (1)

Slow time, (2) MARCH!, when the pupils resume the ordinary step.

ALIGNMENTS.

The instructor first teaches the pupils to align themselves scholar by scholar, the better to comprehend the principles of alignments ; to this end he advances the two men on the right three or more yards, and, having aligned them, commands, (1) *By file,* (2) *Right,* or *Left,* (3) DRESS, (4) Front!

At the command *dress,* the pupils move up successively in quick time, shortening the last step so as to find themselves about six inches behind the alignment. Each pupil then moves on the line, which must never be passed, taking steps of two or three inches, casting his eyes to the right so as to see the buttons on the coat of the pupil second from him, keeping his shoulders square to the front and touching with his elbow that of the one next to him without opening his arms.

At the command *front,* given when the rank is well aligned, the pupils cast their eyes to the front and remain firm.

The pupils having learned to align themselves scholar by scholar, the instructor next aligns the class by the commands, (1) *Right,* or *Left,* (2) DRESS, (3) Front!

At the command *dress,* the entire rank, except the one established as a basis, moves forward and dresses up to the line as previously explained. The instructor verifies the alignment by placing himself at the head of the line and ordering forward or back scholars who are too far to the rear or in advance. This done, he commands, *Front!*

Alignments to the rear are executed on the same principle, the commands being, (1) *Right*, or *Left*, *backward*, (2) DRESS, (3) Front !

Face the pupils to the right. The instructor moves the leading pupil to the right or left, and commands, (1) *Front*, (2) DRESS ! At the command *dress*, the pupils form quickly behind their leader, forming a straight file.

TO MARCH IN LINE.

The class being correctly aligned, the instructor places a well-instructed pupil on the side on which the guide is to be and commands, (1) *Forward*, (2) *Guide right*, or *left*, (3) MARCH !

At the command *march*, the pupils step off smartly with the left foot, the guide marching straight to the front.

The instructor observes in marching in line that the pupils touch lightly the elbow toward the side of the guide; that they open out neither arm ; that they yield to pressure coming from the side of the guide and resist pressure coming from the opposite direction, and that they keep the head direct to the front, no matter on which side the guide may be.

TO MARCH BY THE FLANK.

Being at a halt, the instructor commands, (1) *Right*, or *Left*, (2) FACE ! (3) *Forward*, (4) MARCH ! If in march, the instructor commands, (1) *By the right*, or *left*, *flank*, (2) MARCH!

At the command *march*, given as the right foot strikes the ground, advance and plant the left foot, then turn to the right and step off in the new direction with the right foot. In the march by the flank, the scholars cover each other and keep closed to *facing distance*; that is, to such distance that in forming line the elbows will touch.

TO CHANGE DIRECTION IN COLUMN OF FILES.

Being in march, the instructor commands, (1) *Column right*, or *left*, or (1) *Column half-right*, or *-left*, (2) MARCH!

At the command *march*, the leading file faces to the right, or half-right, and is followed by the other files, who face on the same ground.

TO OBLIQUE.

The pupils, being well established in the principles of the direct march, are exercised in marching obliquely. The squad marching in line, the instructor commands, (1) *Right*, or *Left*, *oblique*, (2) MARCH!

At the command *march*, each pupil makes a half-face to the right and then marches straight in the new direction. As the pupils no longer touch elbows they glance along the shoulders of the nearest files, toward the side to which they are obliquing, and regulate their steps so that their shoulders are always behind those of the next pupil on that side and that his head conceals the heads of the other pupils in the rank. The pupils preserve the same length of pace and the same degree of obliquity; **the line of** the rank remaining parallel to its original position.

To resume the original direction the instructor commands, (1) *Forward*, (2) MARCH!

WHEELINGS.

A wheel is a circular movement by which the front of a squad, set of fours, company, etc., is placed at right angles to its original position, or changes ninety degrees.

An about is a circular movement by which the front of a squad, set of fours, company, etc., is placed facing to the rear or changed one hundred and eighty degrees.

Wheelings are of two kinds: on fixed and on movable pivots.

WHEELING ON A FIXED PIVOT.

Being at a halt the instructor commands, (1) *In circle, right*, or *left, wheel*, (2) MARCH!

At the command *march*, the pupils, except the pivot-man, step off with the left foot, turning at the same time the head a little to the left, the line of the eyes of the pupils to their left; the pivot-man marks time strictly in his place, gradually turning his body, to conform to the movement of the marching flank; the pupil who conducts this flank takes steps of twenty inches, and, from the first step, advances the left shoulder a little, casts his eyes along the rank, and feels lightly the elbow of the next pupil toward the pivot, but never pushes him.

' The other pupils touch with the elbow toward the pivot, resist pressure from the opposite side, conform to the movement of the marching flank, and shorten their steps according to their distance from it. After wheeling around the circle several times the instructor commands, (1) *Squad*, (2) HALT!

WHEELING ON A MOVABLE PIVOT.

Being in march, to change direction the instructor commands, (1) *Right*, or *Left*, *wheel*, (2) MARCH, (3) *Forward*, (4) MARCH!

The first command is given when the class is three yards from the wheeling-point.

At the command *march*, the wheel is executed as on a fixed pivot, except that the pivot-man, instead of turning in his place, takes steps of nine inches, and thus gains ground forward in describing a small curve so as to clear the wheeling-point.

The radius of the circle described by the pivot-man increases with the size of the class, and is equal to nearly one half of the front of the squad or subdivision.

Wheelings on fixed or movable pivot being important movements, the instructor requires the pupils successively to act as pivots and to conduct the marching flank.

TO FORM COLUMN OF FOURS FROM COLUMN OF TWOS OR FILES.

(See Fig. **1**.)

Marching in column **of twos the** teacher commands, (1) *Form fours,* (2) **Left,** or *Right, oblique,* (3) MARCH! At the command **march, the** leading two of each **four** take the short step ; the rear two oblique to the left until they uncover the leading **two, when** they **resume** the forward march. Having formed **column of files** from column of twos or fours, to form column of fours **the** teacher commands, (1) *Form fours,* (2) *Left,* or *Right, oblique,* (3) MARCH! At the command *march,* number one of the first four **moves forward** three yards **and halts ; the** other **files of** the first four **oblique to** the left **and** place themselves successively on the left of the leading file ; **the** other fours **success-** ively form as explained for the first, the leading **file of** each halting **at** about sixty inches from the correspond- ing file **of the four next** in front.

Column of Twos is formed from column of **files on the** same principles. (See Fig. **2.**)

In forming column of fours, **or twos, the teacher** commands, **Left,** or *Right, oblique,* **according as the** right or left is in **front.**

TO FORM COLUMN OF TWOS FROM LINE.

The teacher **commands,** (1) *Twos, right,* or *left,* (2) MARCH! **The two wheel** to the right on **numbers one** and three of each **four as** pivots, and **to** the left **on** numbers two and four. The column of twos is **formed**

Fɪɢ. 1

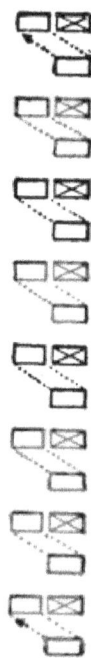

Fɪɢ. 2.

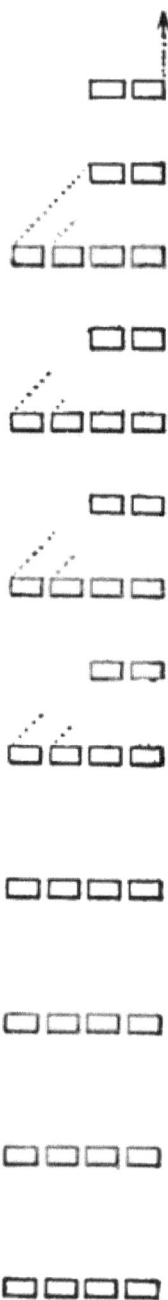

Fɪɢ. 3.

18

in line by the commands, (1) *Twos left*, or *right*, (2)
MARCH! (3) *Guide right*, or *left ;* or, (3) *Company*, (4)
HALT! (5) *Right*, or *Left*, (6) DRESS, (7) FRONT! The
line is formed to the *left* or *right*, according as the
right or left is in front.

TO FORM COLUMN OF FILES FROM LINE.

The teacher commands, if at a halt, (1) *Right*, or
Left, (2) FACE ; (3) *Forward*, (4) MARCH! If in march :
(1) *By the right*, or *left, flank*, (2) MARCH!

TO FORM COLUMN OF TWOS OR FILES FROM COLUMN OF FOURS.

(See Fig. 3.)

The teacher commands, (1) *Right*, or *Left, by twos*,
(2) MARCH! At the second command, the two files on
the right of each four move forward in quick time ;
the two files on the left mark time till disengaged,
when they oblique to the right and follow the right
files, keeping closed to facing distance.

Being at a halt, to form column of files the teacher
commands, (1) *Right*, or *Left, by file*, (2) MARCH! At
the command *march*, the right file of the leading four
moves forward, followed in succession by the files on
its left ; when the left file of the leading four is about
to commence to oblique, the right file of the second
four moves to the front, and so on to the rear of the
column, the pupils keeping closed as nearly as possible to facing distance. If marching, the leading file
continues the march, the others halt and resume the

march at the proper **time.** *Column* **of files,** from column **of** twos, is similarly executed.

In forming **column of** twos (or files) the teacher commands, *right,* or *left,* by twos (or by file), according as the right or **left** is in front.

A column of **twos** (or files) **changes** direction, **is** halted and put in march by the same **commands as a** column of fours.

TO FORM COLUMN OF FOURS FROM LINE.

The teacher **commands, (1)** *Fours, right,* **or** *left,* **(2)** MARCH! (3) Halt! At the second **command each set of fours will** wheel **to the right, No. 1 as** a pivot. **At** the **third command** given, **the** instant the front rank gains the perpendicular to the late line, the scholars will halt, and align themselves toward the marching flank.

TO FORM FOURS IN CIRCLE.

The teacher commands, (1) *Fours, right,* or *left, wheel,* (2) MARCH! The fours complete each arc of ninety degrees simultaneously. The teacher enforces strictly the principles of the fixed pivot, requiring the pupils on the marching flank of each four to take the full step of twenty or twenty-three inches, according to the time, without increasing **or** decreasing the cadence. The fours having wheeled round the circle several times **the** teacher commands: (1) *Company,* (2) HALT! **(3)** *Left,* or *right,* (4) DRESS, (5) FRONT! The command *halt* is given as the fours unite in line or forward march.

TO MARCH IN COLUMN OF FOURS TO THE FRONT.

Being in line the teacher commands, (1) *Right*, or *left, forward*, (2) *Fours right*, or *left*, (3) MARCH. (Fig. 4.) At the command *march*, the right four moves straight to the front, shortening the first three or four steps; the other fours wheel to the right on a fixed pivot; the second four, when its wheel is two thirds completed, wheels to the left on a movable pivot, and follows the first four; the other fours, having wheeled to the right, move forward and wheel to the left on a movable pivot on the same ground as the second.

TO HALT COLUMN OF FOURS AND PUT IT IN MARCH.

The teacher commands, (1) *Company*, (2) HALT! and (1) *Forward*, (2) MARCH!

TO OBLIQUE IN COLUMN OF FOURS, AND TO RESUME THE DIRECT MARCH.

(See Fig. 5.)

The teacher commands, (1) *Right*, or *left, oblique*, (2) MARCH! During the oblique the fours preserve their parallelism; the pupil in each rank of fours on the side toward which the oblique is made is the guide of the rank. The leading guide is the guide of the column when the oblique is toward his flank; when the oblique is toward the opposite flank the guide of the front rank of the leading four is the guide of the

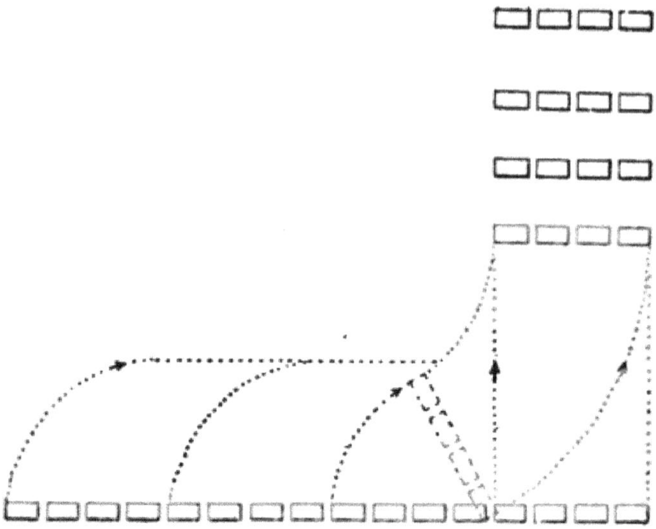

FIG. 4.

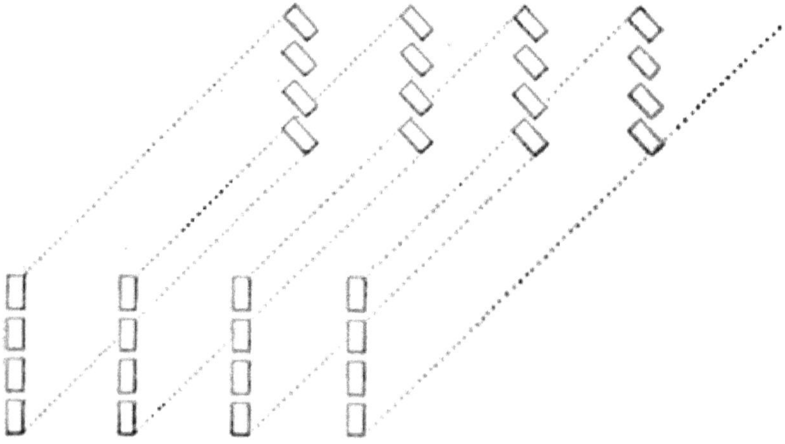

FIG. 5.

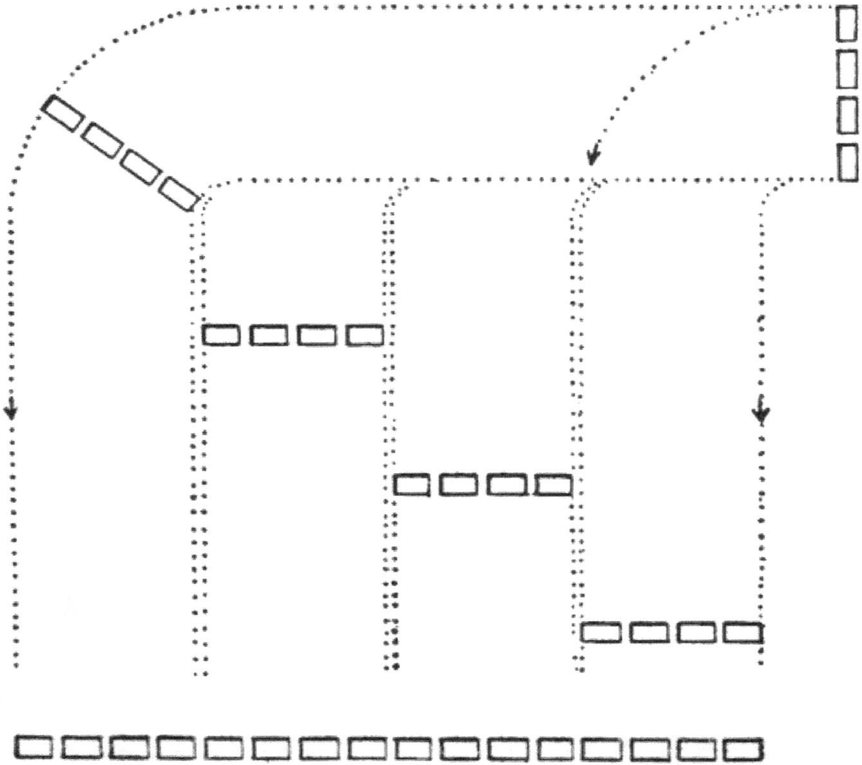

Fig. 7.

Fig. 6.

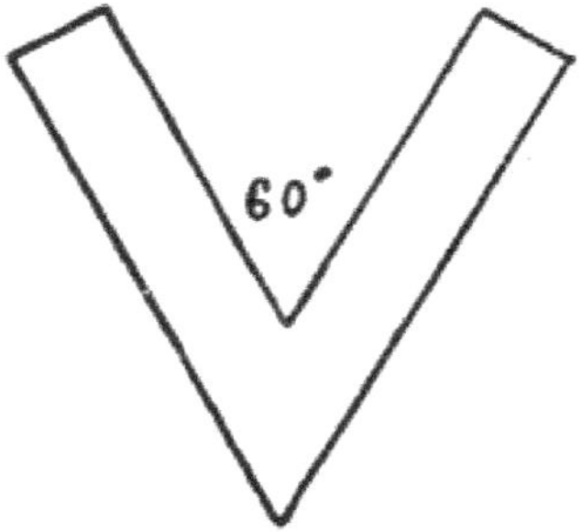

23

column. To resume the direct march the teacher commands, (1) *Forward*, (2) MARCH!

In obliquing a column of fours, or of subdivisions, the guide is always, without indication, on the side toward which the oblique is made; on resuming the direct march the guide, without indication, is on the side it was previous to the oblique. The guides, during the oblique, keep on a line parallel to the original direction. *These rules are general.*

TO CHANGE DIRECTION IN COLUMN OF FOURS.

Being in march, the teacher commands, (1) *Column, right,* or *left,* (2) MARCH! If the change of direction be toward the side of the guide, the guide, at the command *march,* shortens his step and wheels to the right on the arc of a small circle; the leading rank of four wheels on a movable pivot, the pivot-man following in the trace of the guide; if the change of direction be to the side opposite the guide he wheels as if on the marching flank of a rank of four; the wheel being completed, the guide and the leading rank retake the step of twenty inches. The other ranks move forward and wheel on the same ground. *Column half-right,* or *left,* is similarly executed. To put the column of fours in march and change direction at the same time the teacher commands, (1) *Forward,* (2) *Column, right,* or *left,* (3) MARCH! To march the column of fours to the rear the teacher commands, (1) *Fours, right,* or *left, about,* (2) MARCH! The fours wheel about on a fixed pivot.

TO FORM LINE FROM COLUMN OF FOURS.
TO THE RIGHT OR LEFT.

The teacher commands, (1) *Fours right*, or **left**, (2) March! (3) *Guide right*, or *left;* or, (3) *Company*, (4) Halt! (5) *Left*, or *right*, (6) Dress, (7) Front! At the command *march*, the fours wheel to the right on a fixed pivot.

ON THE RIGHT OR LEFT.

(See Fig. 6.)

The teacher commands, (1) *On right*, or *left*, *into line*, (2) March! (3) *Company*, (4) Halt, (5) *Right*, or *left*, (6) Dress, (7) Front! At the command *march*, the leading four wheels to the right on a movable pivot, and moves forward, dressing to the right; the other fours march a distance equal to their front beyond the wheeling-point of the four next preceding, wheel to the right and advance as explained for the first four. At the command *halt*, given when the leading four has advanced company distance in the new direction, it halts, and at the sixth command, given immediately after, dresses to the right; the other fours halt and dress successively upon arriving in line. At the seventh command, given when the last four completes its dressing, all the pupils cast their eyes to the front. In these movements where it is prescribed that the leading four, or subdivision, moves company distance to the front and then halts, the leading four, or subdivision, may be halted at a less distance when necessary. *This rule is general.*

TO FORM TWO RANKS.

To form two ranks from a line of files, the teacher commands, *In two ranks form company*, MARCH ! At the second command the scholar in front will right or left face, the second scholar marches up and back of No. 1 and stands back of him, the third scholar marches alongside of No. 1, the fourth scholar marches up and crosses over back of No. 3, the fifth scholar alongside of No. 3, the sixth back of No. 3, the remaining scholars close in quick time and form alternately front and back.

ALIGNMENTS.

The classes can be quickly aligned or arranged according to height by picking from the class the tallest member, standing him at a little distance from the rest, and then placing the scholars according to their height back of him.

If classes are too small to work with fours, in many cases twos can perform the work of fours.

CHAPTER II.

A ROOM 50 by 35 feet will accommodate about 90 scholars if the foot-marks are placed 6 feet apart, but it is more desirable that the distance should be 7 feet. If scholars are to work several times a week, much time can be saved by the use of foot-marks, which should be arranged according to the diagram. Fig. 7 shows one third the size of a foot-mark. The two lines which form an angle of 60 degrees should be 4 inches long and three quarters of an inch wide.

By placing tracing-paper over the diagram the size or angle can be transferred to a piece of card-board from which a stencil can be cut. It is a good plan to mark on the floor a running track and measure its distance in blocks or parts of a mile.

A line crossing the track should designate the starting and finishing point see Fig. 8. For marking the floor use ladies' shoe-dressing.

DUMB-BELLS.

For children use the one-half or three-quarter pound bell; for adults use the one or two pound bell.

A bell that weighs one pound will do for strong men if the exercise is vigorous.

27

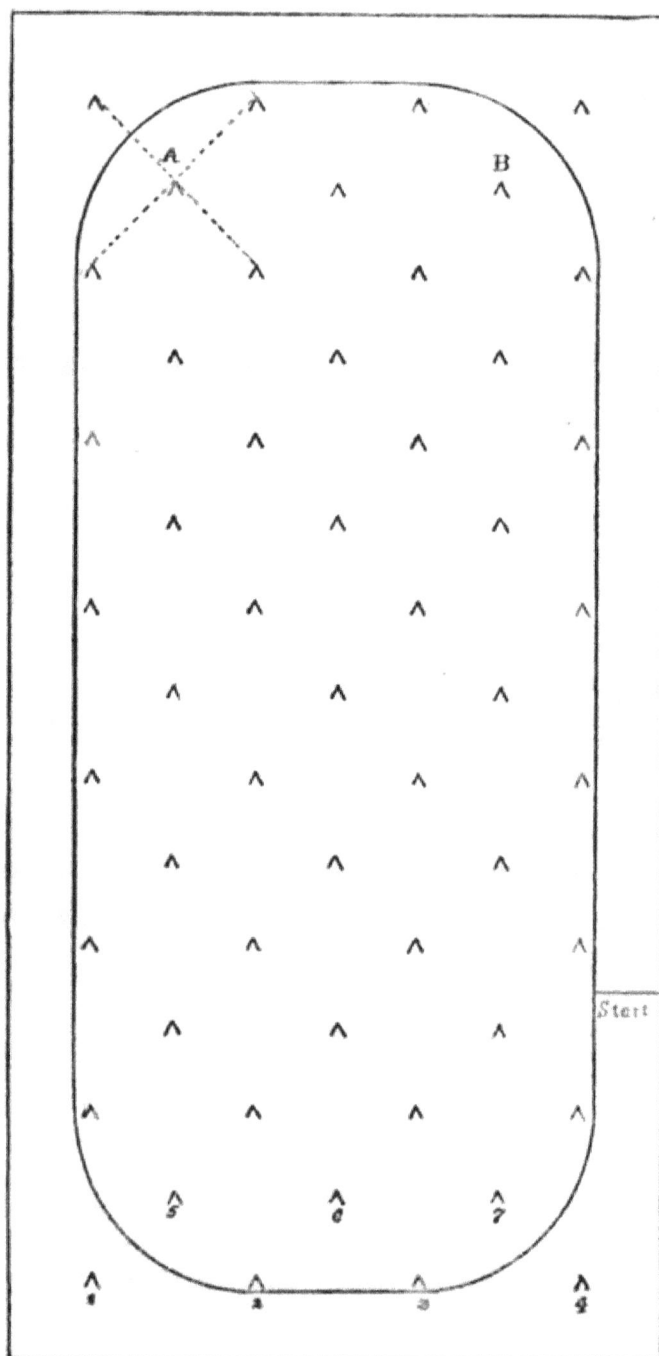

FIG. 8.

28

WANDS.

Use two kinds, one four feet six inches long and three quarters of an inch in diameter for the Manual of Arms and Bayonet drill.

For other exercises the "dowels" furnished by hardware stores will do. They are three feet in length and of any desired diameter: five eighths inch is preferable.

CLUBS.

Use two sizes, one and two pounds. The Author has found that the one-pound club is not too heavy for children between the ages of seven and ten. A two-pound club is heavy enough for men.

POLES.

See page 164 for details.

RACKS.

Bells and clubs should be suspended from wooden racks which are placed around the sides of the room about four feet from the floor. The racks should be made from hard-wood boards 5 inches wide and 1 inch thick. In this, grooves are cut every 6 inches. They should be two inches deep, one inch wide, and beveled at the part near the center of the board, that the bell or club will not so easily fall out (Fig. 9). If by accident the grooves are cut too wide and the clubs slip through, small strips of leather or rubber may be tacked in.

Racks of this kind should be supported by iron knees or brackets. Cast-iron racks are not a success; they break too easily.

For wands, use a box 3 feet high, 18 inches wide, and 2 feet long. This can be divided into compartments for different-sized wands, as desired.

It is important that all light gymnastic appliances be so arranged that they can be taken and replaced quickly. It is not desirable that racks be used for wands.

HOW TO MARK THE FLOOR.

It is quite as hard to tell how to mark the floor as it is to mark it; but a few directions may be of service. Three persons can accomplish this better than two, as two are required to handle the tape while the third marks the floor with chalk. Make the outside lines at least 3 feet from the side of the house. Next arrange that the marks shall be as near 7 feet apart from right to left as the space will permit. Foot-marks nearer than 6 feet prevent certain exercises with the clubs and long wands. Now lay off the lines of foot-marks, 1, 2, 3, 4 (Fig. 8). If the classes are not large, these marks will be sufficient; but if there are more pupils than the number of marks, then make the alternate rows 5, 6, 7.

An easy way to get the distance of the alternate marks is this: Draw intersecting lines at A and B; also at 5 and 7. Hold one end of the tape at A and the other at B, and mark off the intervening space. Do the same at 5 and 7. Now hold one end of the

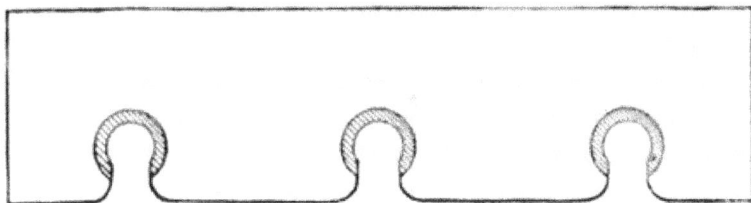

FIG. 9.

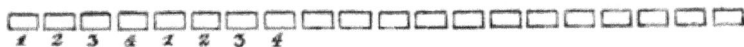

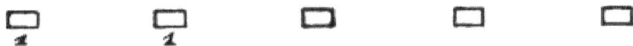

FIG. 10.

tape **at A and the** other at 5, mark **off** the space
between. Continue this for the other lines. When
the preliminary chalk-marks are made, notice whether
the lines are straight from front to rear, right to left,
and in the **oblique** directions. If they are, take the
cardboard stencil and mark the floor with ink, paint,
or liquid shoe-blacking.

FOOT-MARKS.

It frequently happens **that** a class will have **to exer-**
cise **in a** room where there **are** no foot-marks. **In this**
case it will **be** well to know of **several** methods of placing scholars **on** the floor, **that the** class may present a
uniform appearance.

One method is illustrated **by** Fig. **10.** A row of
scholars is represented facing **in** the direction of the
arrow; the class **is** supposed **to have** been numbered 1,
2, 3, 4, **1, 2,** 3, 4, etc., and that each scholar knows his
number. The command is given *Company, front, open*
files, four paces, MARCH! In which case each pupil **will**
multiply his own number by the number of **paces**
given in the command. He will then take that number
of steps straight to the front at the command *March.*
When the various positions have been taken, **it** will be
found that No. 1 has taken four paces **to** the front, No.
2 eight paces, **No. 3** twelve, and No. **4** sixteen paces.
The arrangement seen **in** Fig. 10 shows the position
of the scholars when the command has been executed.

To bring the pupils back to a line, give the command
Front, close files, MARCH! at which command No. **4**

stands still, while 1, 2, and 3 march to the front until they are in line with No. 4.

It is not necessary in performing this evolution that the class count fours or that they take four paces to the front. They can count threes, fives, or sixes, and they can take three, five, or six paces to the front according to the wish of the teacher; but in any case the pupil should multiply his number by the number of paces given, and should take that number of steps to the front.

FOOT-MARKS—SECOND METHOD.

In Fig. 11, the line *AB* represents a file of scholars marching in the direction of the arrow *C*. No. 1 turns to the left and marches in the direction of the arrow *D*; he is followed by Nos. 2, 3, 4, 5, and 6, who fall back from each other about five or six paces. When the first six files have marched the required distance, they execute a left face, and march in the direction of the arrow *E*; they are followed in turn by the second six files, and so on until all of the original file of pupils have opened order and are marching in the direction of the arrow *E*. The teacher gives the command *Halt;* when the first six have marched to the front of the hall, the other sixes will stop at any specified number of paces from the six next in front of them. To bring the pupil back to single file, give the command *right face, forward, close order,* MARCH; when Nos. 2, 3, 4, 5, and 6 will march up back of No. 1, in which case the first set can march in any given direction, to be followed by the others in their turn.

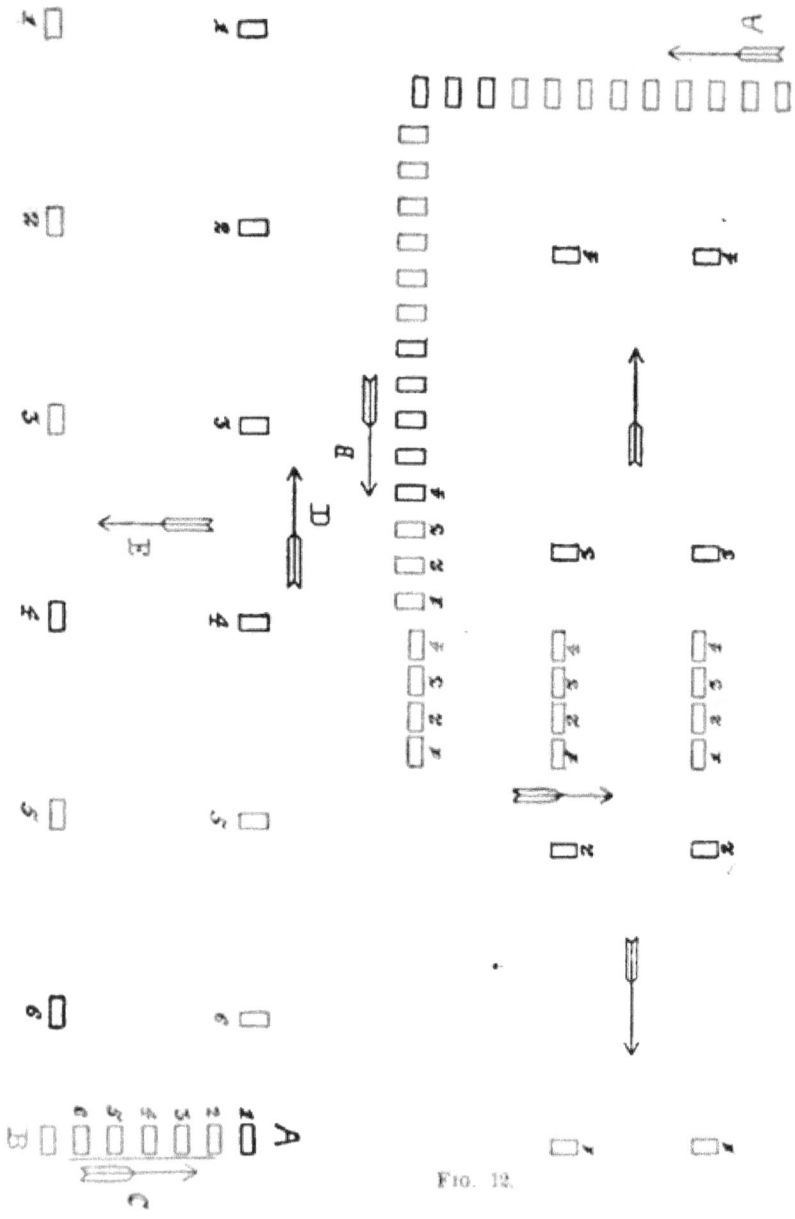

Fig. 11.

Fig. 12.

34

This method of taking places on the floor will require practice.

FOOT-MARKS—THIRD METHOD.

Fig. 12 represents the third method of taking positions for exercises. It represents a file of pupils marching in the direction of the arrows *A* and *B*. The first four executes a left flank movement and marches in the direction of the arrow *C*. When they have gone a specified distance, 1 and 2 right face, 3 and 4 left face ; 1 and 4 take 9 steps and 2 and 3 take 3 steps in the direction they face.

They are followed in turn by the other fours, who execute the same manœuver but stop 6 paces from the four in front of them.

When all have taken their places, they face front.

To bring the pupils back to a line of fours, command, *Company*, Face! At the command *face*, 1 and 2 left face and 3 and 4 right face. *Close order*, March! At the command *march*, the pupils march up to form a four, then front face.

In the methods described, it is not essential that the intervals in marching or the number of steps be always the same. The teacher must use his own discretion, and govern the distance by the size of the room and the number in the class.

CHAPTER III.

MUSCULAR DEVELOPMENT.

THE immediate results of gymnastic exercise are apparent in the muscular system. We give an exercise a stated number of times, that it may produce, as a result, an increase in the quality and size of the muscle.

We know that exercise will do this. The next step is, Which muscles shall we use most? how frequently shall they be used? and how long at a time?

These questions can not be answered until the common physical defects caused by our use or our development of certain muscles, are known. These we shall investigate. Teachers will notice that, in the routine work and play of pupils, they use one part of the body more than another; consequently this part not only receives a greater share of development, but it is apparent by the defect it causes. The physical imperfections spoken of in this chapter are caused principally by muscular contraction. They are not organic; that is, they do not include disease of any internal organs.

A few statements will make this chapter more intelligible.

1. Muscles are made up of fibers; these in turn are

36

composed of fibrils, which owe their existence to a combination of individual elements or cells.

2. **Use of a** muscle causes the destruction of these **cells, which are at once carried off** by the blood **while** · **new elements take their place.**

3. Rapid **use of a muscle causes** rapid **change in** its tissue, **which in turn necessitates a quick flow of** blood to carry off the **old and** leave new **cells.** This accounts for the accelerated beating of **the heart in exercise.**

4. **Blood** must be purified **by** coming in contact **with the air in the** lungs before it can **repair** tissue. **Any change in the speed** of its current produces **a corresponding** change in the action of **the lungs. This accounts for the rapid** breathing **of pupils after exer**cising.

5. The blood **receives the constructive** elements, or cells, **from bodily nourishment. If the exercise is too** violent, the repair **cannot keep pace with it and a pupil** experiences fatigue.

6. When the blood **has** entirely absorbed the **con**structive element from the **store of** nourishment, it is necessary that there **be a new supply of aliment.** We can consequently understand why exertion **causes** hunger.

7. A muscle **is always ready for immediate** action. **It is** stretched to **such** a degree **that** no time is required to tighten **it before it** will do **its** work. Moreover, a muscle is contracted in proportion **to its** size. This fact **will** account **for some of the** defects we shall speak **of later.**

The author, in his teaching, has used simple illus-
trations or diagrams, to prove this to children ; the result being that they more easily comprehend for what

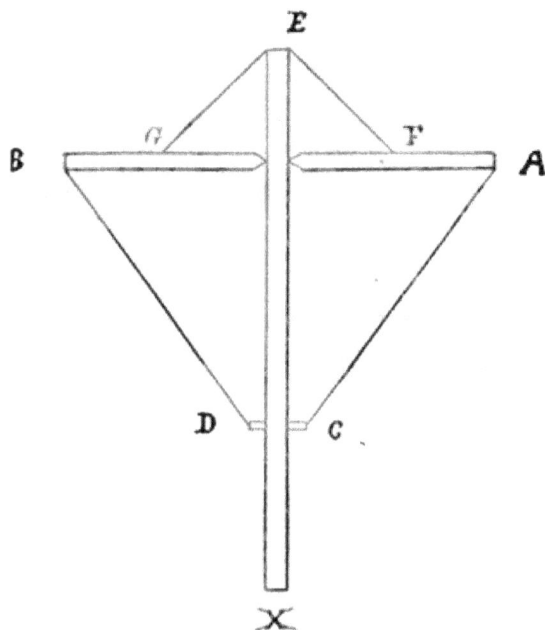

Fig. 13.—Rear view of a well-built boy.

they are striving, and they **work with a better** understanding of the "how and **why.**"

The diagrams used **are** crude, but they serve the
purpose.

The diagram in Fig. 13 will illustrate the statement
in No. 7.

The line **X** represents the back, *A* the right, and *B*
the left shoulder ; *AC* are muscles going from the right
shoulder down to the back; *BD*, corresponding muscles
on **the** left.

In a child whose muscles are of the same strength on both the right and left sides, the shoulders will be even, as in Fig. 13ª; but if the right side is more used than the left, as it generally is, the muscles on that side are stronger, they contract with more force than those on the left, and draw the right shoulder down, as in Fig. 14. Not only this, but they tend to draw the part of the spine to which they are attached out of

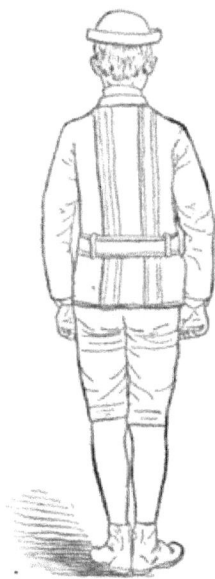

Fig. 13a.

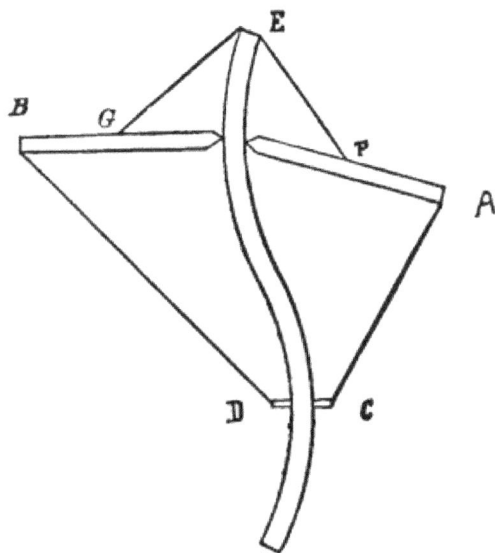

Fig. 14.

a plumb line, producing what physicians call a lateral curve of the spine. See Fig. 15ª.

Fig. 14 shows the outline of the back of a pupil who has over-developed his right side. The application may be partly seen in Fig. 15.

The treatment of this defect is simple. Develop the muscles *EF*, *EG*, *BD*. The muscles *EG*, and *EF*, above the shoulders, may be strengthened by,—

1. Shrugging the shoulders.
2. Swinging the right arm from the side up.

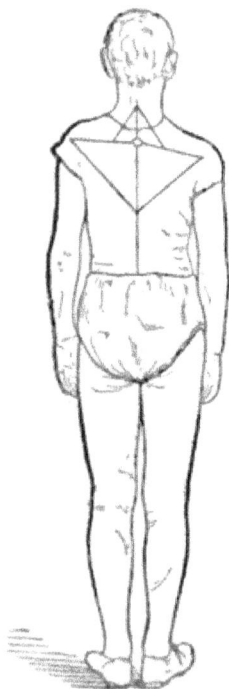 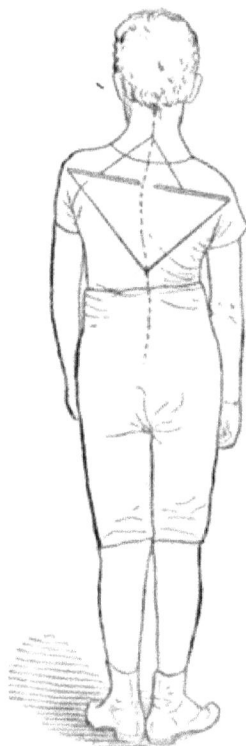

FIG. 15.   FIG. 15a.

FIG. 15.—Defect. Right shoulder lower than the left, caused by over-development of the right side.

FIG. 15a shows uneven shoulders and a lateral curve in the spine. Caused by resting the weight of the body on one leg.

3. Thrusting the arm up.
4. Bending the head forcibly to the right.

These rules are general and apply **to the muscles** on the left also.

The muscles *BD* may be developed by,—

1. Forcing the shoulder down, the opposite of shrugging.

2. Thrusting the arms down.

3. Striking the hands below the waist **in front and** back of the body.

The chest muscles are **used** more than **the** corresponding muscles **of** the back. The arms perform duties more in front than back of the body, with this **result :** the **chest** muscles are the stronger, **and, so,** draw the shoulders forward, producing " **round shoulders."** The chest muscles on the right **side, being** stronger, **not only** draw the shoulders down, **but also** forward. **As** these muscles are connected with **the** upper and outward angle of the shoulder-blade, they draw that forward ; this throws the lower **inner angle** out, giving it an undue prominence,—at the **same time a** deformity so common **among young women, called** " wings."

To overcome this, develop **the muscles** between the shoulders. This is done best by any motion that will bring the shoulder-blades together. Remember this. To overcome such defects by exercise, teach the pupil to **take the** correct **position.** To do this, he will call into action the very muscles you wish to develop. For instance, tell **a** round-shouldered boy **to throw his** shoulders **back ; at** the same time show him how. If he does it properly, he has taken,

unconsciously perhaps, the best method there is for cur-
ing that particular trouble ; and this same
movement should be given as an exercise.

Require a pupil whose head drops down
forward to force it back to the normal
position. By doing this rightly, he will
use the very muscles you are anxious to
strengthen. See series No. 3, Free Gymnastics.

The Head.—Fig. 16 represents a side
view of a pupil. *X* is the back or spine,
A the head, *HG* the front and *IG* the
back muscles. The head is bent forward
or turned to the right and left, looking
down oftener than back and up. The
muscles *HG*, which draw the head forward, are stronger than those, *IG*, which
force it back. This produces the most
common of the physical defects, "a drooping head." See Fig. 17.

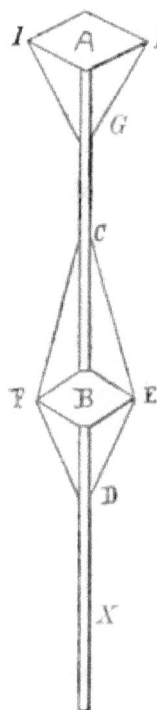

Fig. 16.

Teachers should take into consideration
the action of the small cushions between the different
parts of the spine. If they become permanently compressed in front, they will not spring the bones back.

To draw the head back, develop the muscles *IG*
on the posterior neck. This is done,—

1. By bending the head back ;

2. By turning the face obliquely up to the right and
left ;

3. Keeping the head upright, try to touch the chin
to the throat.

For the application of diagram No. 17 to the head, see Fig. 18.

Fig. 19 shows a sloping or "bottle-necked" youth, with lower left shoulder.

Hips.—If the teacher will stand at the head of a line of raw recruits, and look down it, one of the

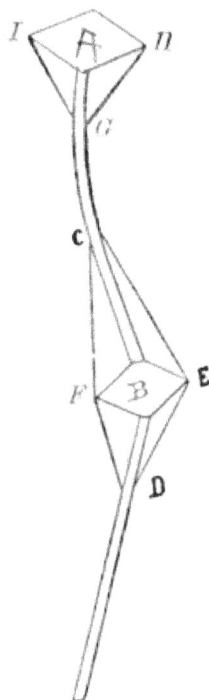

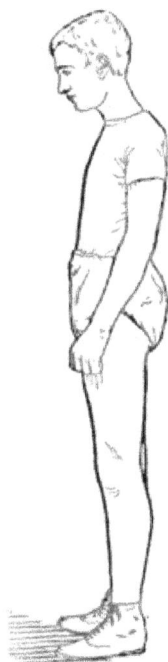

Fig. 17.   Fig. 18.

Fig. 18.—Drooping head and flat chest.

most noticeable things will be the undue prominence of the "stomachs." They project farther forward than the chest. This is a defect that can be
remedied by forcing the hips back. It is common to

boys and girls. The strong muscles which connect the lower back and hips are constantly in use when one is standing, walking, and, sometimes, sitting. They correspond to CF in Fig. 17, and are much stronger than the front muscles, CE. The muscles

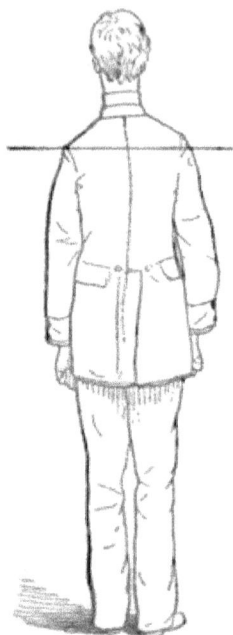
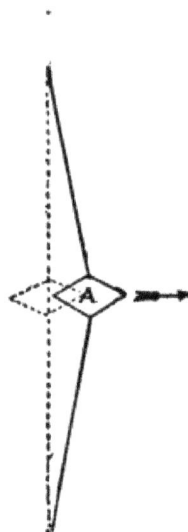

Fig. 19.　　　　　Fig. 20.

Fig. 19.—A bottle-necked youth. It is impossible in this style of illustration to show the defect as seen in the photograph.

DF, which connect the hips and back upper thigh, are also very powerful, as they should be; otherwise, the body would topple forward. But pupils do not strengthen the muscles EC as much as they should; consequently, the combined action of CF and DF is greater than EC and ED, the result being that the

hips are thrown too far forward, as seen in Fig. 20. The
dotted lines show the correct position. The remedy
lies in strengthening the muscles *EC* and *ED*. This
can be done by flexing the thighs, (see page 64); bending
the body well forward, trying to touch the hands to

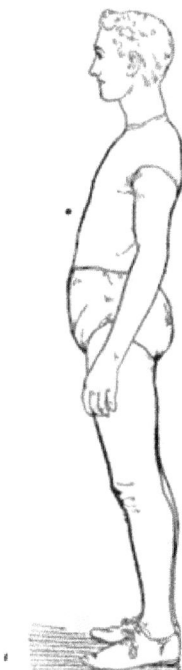

FIG. 21.—Projecting hips.   FIG. 22.—Side view of a well-built boy.

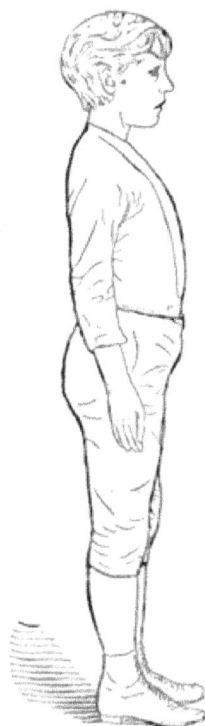

the floor; or by forcing back, and keeping back, the
hips. The author has noticed among some fashion-
able pupils, boys particularly, a defect just the opposite of the one described. There is a bend in the
body, the hips are thrown so far back and the

shoulders **so far forward** that the boy has the appearance of imitating the "Grecian bend." What is at first merely affectation, finally becomes habit. A boy who stands erect (see Fig. 22) can be compared to a straight post, which will sustain an enormous weight; but the boy who does **not** stand erect **is** like a much **larger** post that is bent, and which **will not** bear **so much**

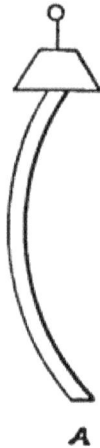 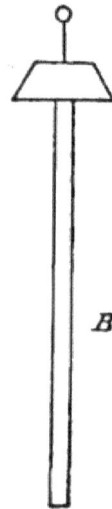

A

Fig. 23.　　　　　　　Fig. 24.

weight **as** the straight **one.** This **can** be illustrated by placing a small piece of iron on **a** toothpick that is straight: now bend the toothpick, when it will be **seen** that it can **not** sustain the pressure it did formerly (Figs. 23 and **24**).

The Waist.—The weak spot in our pupils is here. A narrow waist cannot be a strong one; a deep one **is** not desirable. By the waist, we mean that part of the trunk adjacent to the thorax and hips. A wide waist can be obtained by any exercise which will widen the thorax, which see ; also by bending and rolling the trunk in any direction.

The Thorax.—Special attention should be given to the development of this portion of the trunk. It contains the heart and lungs ; therefore it should not be cramped or unduly compressed, as these vital organs would suffer by any such restriction.

The defective thorax is found to be **too narrow at its base.** It is enough if we can increase the length of the diameters in this vicinity. This can be done by breathing-exercises, which see ; or by any effort that will cause deep breathing ; by any motion where the hands are raised from the side forcibly above the head ; by bending the head or body back ; by forcing the elbows back ; by swinging the rigid arms, held shoulder-high, from front to rear ; by placing the hands on the hips and forcing the chest forward and the head and hips back.

The Arm.—The fore-arm is generally better developed, in proportion, than the upper arm. This is because the hand and fingers are used more than the upper arm. To develop the front upper arm, take any motion that will bring the hand to the shoulder.

The back upper arm : Any motion that will force the hand from the shoulder or chest, or extend the flexed arm in any direction.

Front fore-arm : **Shut the hands tight, flex the hand on the fore-arm.**

Back fore-arm : Open forcibly the closed hand ; extend the flexed hand.

The Leg.—The inside of the upper leg is not, as a rule, well developed. The muscles running down the front upper leg **are much** stronger and larger than the corresponding muscles on the back upper leg. **This** we expect, but the back upper leg can and **should** be better developed than **it** is. (We are speaking now of the muscles which run from the upper **to** the lower leg.) As the foot and leg **are used** more than the thigh, the leg is better developed **and** larger in proportion.

To develop the thigh :

Front : Raise and lower the body (Fig. **42) ; take** any running, jumping, or hopping exercise.

Back : Flex the leg ; take running exercises.

Inside : Swing, charge, or **step one leg** across in front or **back** of the other.

Back (calf) : Raising on the toes, raising and lowering the body, running, jumping, hopping, and fast walking.

Front : Any motion that raises the toes from the floor ; fast walking.

Ankle.—All leg motions strengthen the ankle.

To recapitulate, we find the following common physical defects that may **be** helped by **light** gymnastics :

HEAD . . . . . . { drops **forward** ;
carried a little to one side ;
chin raised **too** high.

SHOULDERS. . { round, stooping, sloping, and uneven ;
one lower than the other.

THORAX..... { one side better developed than the other ;
the diameters at the base too short ;

UPPER BACK { right shoulder-blade too prominent in right-handed people.

SPINE........ { side or lateral curves ;
bends too far forward from between the shoulders.

WAIST....... { too narrow ;
abdominal muscles weak.

HIPS .... { thrown too far forward.

ARMS ...... { fore-arm better developed than the up-per arm.

LEG .... { better developed than thigh.

THIGH ..... { inside and back poorly developed.

The diagrams on pages **50** and **51** will illustrate the location of sets of muscles. It will not only make **more** intelligible the chapter **that treats** of defects, **their cause** and treatment, but **also the article on the develop-ment of** various portions **of the muscular system.**

LOCATION OF SETS OF MUSCLES.

In **Fig. 25,** the line,—
1. Indicates the front of the **neck ;**
2. The **turn** of the shoulder ;
3. The chest ;
4. The front upper arm ;
5. The front fore-arm ;
6. The front thigh ;
7. The front leg ;

8. The waist (between *A* and *B*);
9. The ankle.

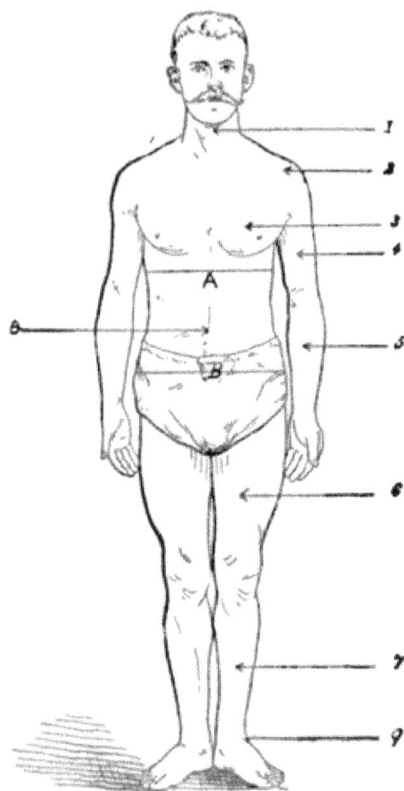

Fig. 25.—Location of sets of muscles, front view.

In Fig. 26, the line,—
1. Indicates the back neck
2. The upper back (between *A* and *B*);
3. The back upper arm ;
4. The lower back ;
5. The back fore-arm ;

6. The back thigh ;
7. The calf ;
8. The inside thigh ;

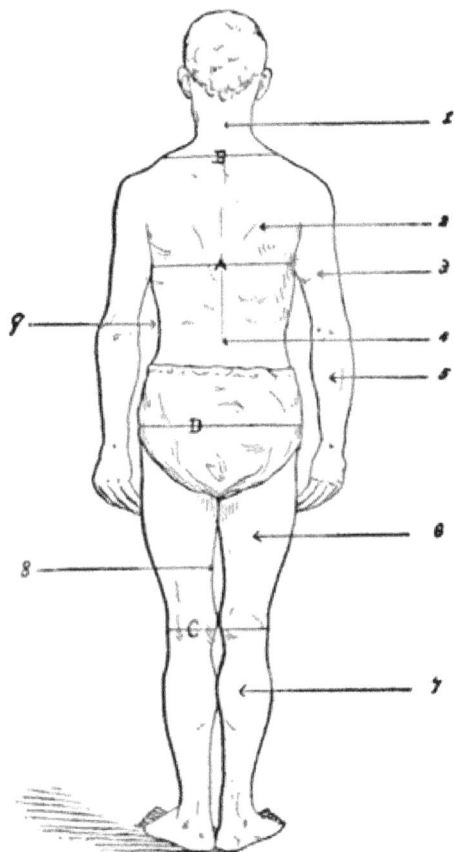

Fig. 26.—Location of sets of muscles, back view.

9. The side of the waist.

The thigh extends from *D* to *C* ; the leg from *C* down.

The diagram, **Fig. 27,** shows the direction in which such motions as stepping, thrusting, charging, etc., can be made.

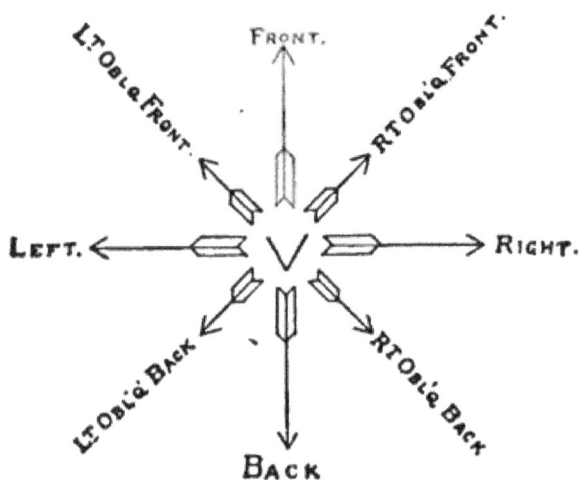

FIG. 27.

Diagonal and oblique directions **are the same.**

POSITIONS.

In executing the exercises given in the Manual, **the** rigid arms may be held with the hands,—

1. **At** the side or DOWN (Fig. 28);
2. Shoulder-high **to the side,** or OUT;
3. Above the head, or UP;
4. Shoulder-high front, or FRONT;
5. Hip-high to the front and side;
6. Head-high to **the** front or side. (In No. 6, the hands are a little higher than the head.)
7. **The** hands may be held obliquely front, hip-high, head-high, and shoulder-high.

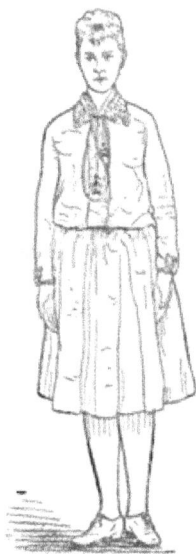

FIG. 28.
Position of a soldier.

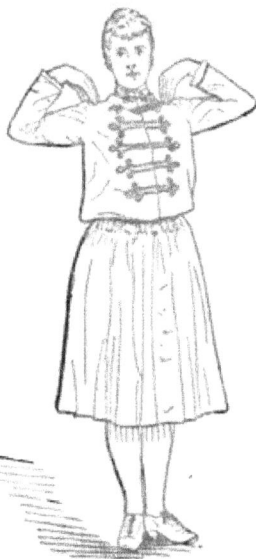

FIG. 29.
Hands on shoulders.

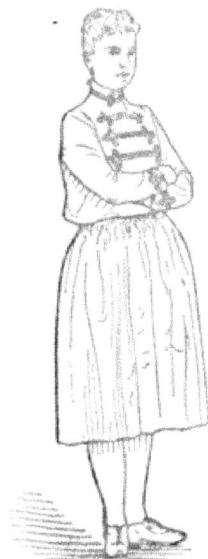

FIG. 31.
Arms folded in front.

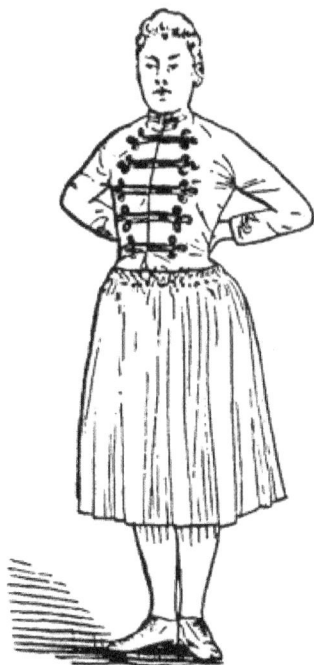

FIG. 30.
Hands on the hips.

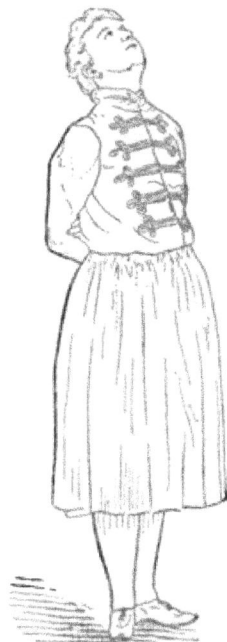

FIG. 32.
Bending the head backward.

8. By bending **the** arms. The hands **may be** held elbow-high to the **front, on** the chest, shoulders (Fig. 29), and hips (Fig. 30).

9. The hands may **be** clasped in front **and back,** on the head, back of **the** neck.

10. The arms may **be** folded **in** front (Fig. 31) and **back** (Fig. 32).

CHAPTER IV.

Nearly all exercises that can be used in light gymnastics are made up of one or more of the following motions, or some combination of them.

They bear the same relation to the series taught in this book, that the alphabet does to words. They are called the A, B, C's of light gymnastics.

If pupils are well drilled in these simple motions, it will be as easy a matter to put them together as it is for a child to spell a short word after it has mastered its letters.

It is of course necessary that they be well learned.

THE LIGHT GYMNASTIC ALPHABET.

1 Stepping
2 Charging ;
3 Lunging ;
4 Hopping ;
5 Running ;
6 Swaying ;
7 Swinging ;
8 Turning or twisting ;
9 Raising or lowering ;
10 Bending or straightening ;
11 Thrusting ;
12 Rolling ;
13 Opening and closing ;
14 Slapping ;
15 Stamping ;
16 Circling ;
17 Percussing ;
18 Shrugging.

A flexing and a bending motion are the same.

Extend and straighten are synonymous.

The alphabet is applied to the various parts of the body as follows :

Neck and Head.—Bending, rolling, and twisting.

Eyes.—Opening, closing, and rolling.

Mouth.—Opening and closing.

Shoulders.—Shrugging and rolling.

Arms.—Thrusting, swinging, circling, flexing, extending, raising, lowering, twisting.

Hands.—Opening, closing, percussing, slapping.

Trunk and Body.—Bending, twisting, rolling.

Legs.—Swinging, raising and lowering, flexing, extending, twisting, stepping, charging, lunging, swaying, hopping, running.

Feet.—Raising toes or heels, twisting.

Abbreviations used : Right—rt. ; left—l. ; foot—ft. ; diagonally—diag.; oblique—oblq.; chest—ch.; shoulder —sh.; high—h.; club—c.; wand—w.; bell—b.; sword —sw.

1. A Stepping Motion is made by swinging the leg in any one of the given directions, and touching the toes lightly to the floor.

The length of a stepping motion is the length of the foot. The object of this exercise is to acquire control of the leg only : there should be no motion to any other part of the body. A class of children, if properly drilled in this exercise, can stand before the table and execute stepping motions, and it will be difficult to tell whether they are moving. A stepping motion is not given to the left wit' the right foot, or to the right with the left foot (Figs. 33 and 34).

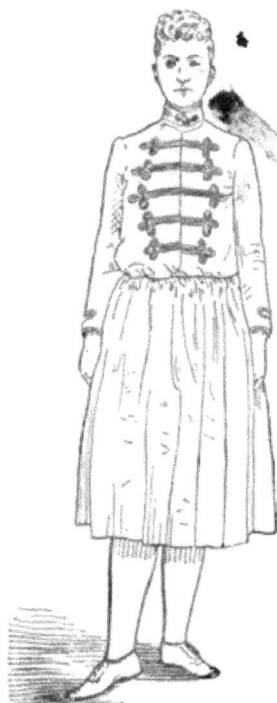 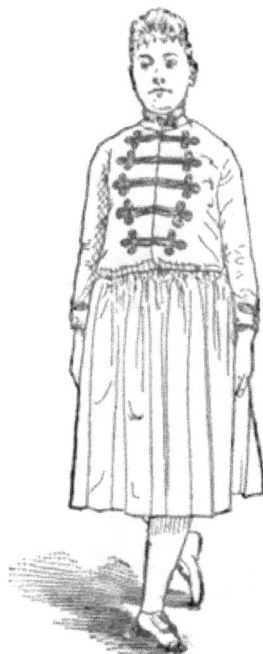

FIG. 33.   FIG. 34.

FIG. 33 —Stepping motion.   Right foot diagonally forward.
FIG. 34.—Stepping motion.   Right foot diagonally back to the left.

2. A **Charging Motion** is made in the same directions as a stepping motion. It consists in throwing the right foot forward twice the length of the foot; the right knee is bent to such a degree that the leg in front is parallel to the back leg. An exception to this is found when charging motions are made with the right foot on the left side ; and to the rear.

The heels of both feet, as well as the toes, must rest on the floor; the back leg should be straight. The knee of the charging leg is a little farther forward than the toes of the same leg; the chest is farther to the front

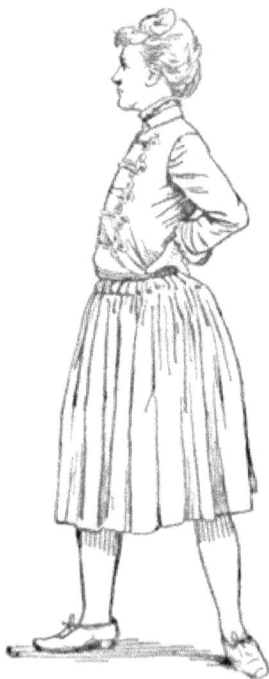

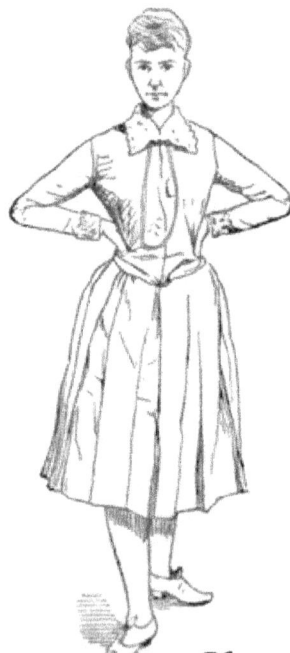

FIG. 85.—Charging motion to the right. FIG. 86.—Charging motion to the front.

than to the hips; while the trunk of the body keeps an upright position. This rule will apply only to the following directions: front, right oblique, and to the right. In the other directions, as far as possible observe the rule. In any charging motion, touch the ball of the foot to the floor first. It will be found that the charging motion is a difficult one to teach (Figs. 35 and 36).

3. **Lunging.**—The lunge is used principally in fencing, and is made in but one direction—to the front. It is about twice the length of a charge. With regard to the general position of the body, the rules for charging apply here. The thigh of the charging leg is parallel to the floor; the heels should be in the same line from front to rear.

4. **Swaying Motions.**—A swaying motion is made to the front, oblique right, and back. To execute it, charge the right foot to the front (see rules for charging motions); now, without changing the position of the feet, shift the weight of the body from the front to the back leg.

This is done by merely straightening the front leg and bending the back leg. The weight of the body can be changed back and forth until the exercise is finished. In a swaying motion, the trunk of the body should be kept in an upright position, the chest always more prominent than the hips. Do not permit the head to drop forward.

5. **A Hopping Motion** is executed on one leg. It consists in leaping lightly from the floor, two or three inches up and down, alighting and starting from the same foot. The knee should always be bent in alighting. The hands in this exercise should be placed on the hips. This movement can be varied by allowing the pupils to hop on one or both feet. Hopping from one foot to another, without gaining ground, is the same as running in place. The difference between running and walking is that, in walking, one foot is always on the ground; while running is nothing but a

series of leaps at which time both feet are off the ground.

6. **Running.**—**This** is considered the best of all exercises for developing the capacity and endurance of the lungs, or, as athletes call it, " the wind."

It is an exercise that should be taken every day.

There is danger in permitting pupils to run around a school-room provided with desks, as they are liable to fall while rounding the corners, or to trip over the legs of the desk.

This danger can be obviated by permitting scholars to " run in place," which is the same to running that marking time is to marching. It consists in hopping from one foot to the other without gaining ground.

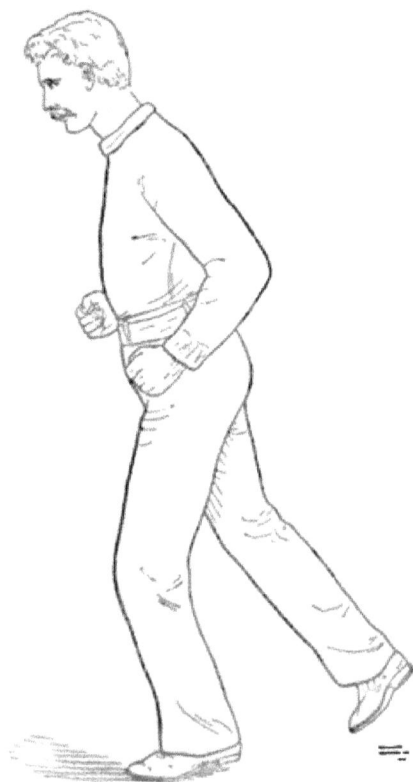

Fig. 37.—Running in place.

When taking this exercise, at the command, *In place!* assume the position described under Double Time (p. 11), or the hands can be placed on the hips; throw the chest forward and the hips back ; keep the head erect. At the command, RUN! raise the left foot from the floor; then spring from the right to the left foot, and from the left to the right foot, and so on until the command, HALT! or SLOW TIME is given.

This brings the count or accent on the left foot, as in marching.

"Running in place" may be executed in four ways. The first or most common consists in throwing the heels back and up to the height of the knee.

In the second and more difficult method, the pupil is to strike the back of the upper thigh with the heel of the foot of the same leg.

The third method is made by throwing the legs sideways, and the fourth by raising the knees up in front.

In this exercise, as in many others, some pupils must be excused or allowed to rest after a brief period of work (from 30 to 60 counts).

If a class is to exercise in a hall where the opportunity for running around the room is given, then it is well to give the pupils a chance to make a circuit of the calistheneum, the girls going in one direction and the boys in another.

A run to music requires practice, but, when correctly done, is a beautiful exercise. The class should practice running in place before making a "course run."

Children, if permitted to stamp the left foot on the first of each four counts, will soon get the time.

Teachers should remember this:

1st. When running, never touch the heels to the floor.

2d. Pupils must keep their **running** distance, which is arm's length from the one in front of them.

3d. Pupils must not try to turn square **corners.**

4th. When pupils are tired and wish to stop, **they must not run** out between the lines. Those in the inside line should **step to the center** of the **room ; those** in the outside **line** should stop in **some corner** or along the side of the room.

5th. **If** the floor **is** slippery, **sprinkle sand** over it.

6th. Do not **force** children to breath through their noses. It looks better **to see closed** mouths ; but the **rule should not be** made **arbitrary. Some** of the best runners breath through their mouths when running.

7th. Do not quicken the **time much above 190 steps** to the minute if **the classes are large.**

A failure on the teacher's part **to explain** or enforce **the above** rules, may result in **a serious** accident **to some member of** the class.

The writer has adopted **this method, and** finds **it** quite satisfactory.

At the beginning **of the** year, once or twice a **week** the class runs from one to two blocks, **the** track on the floor indicating **the** distance. The course is **gradually** increased until spring, when the entire class can **safely** run from three quarters **to one** and one-half **miles.** Pupils, when **tired,** are allowed to drop out ; but any scholar who has **a** side-ache, or who experiences any unpleasant results from a long run, and does not drop **out,** is barred from the class **the next** run if this can **be** ascertained.

In the long run, **it is** not necessary **for** the scholars to work with music, nor is it essential that they should keep step, providing they keep their distance.

7. **Swinging Motions** are applicable to both the arms and legs, and are made by swinging the leg, without bending the knee, in one of the given directions; and it

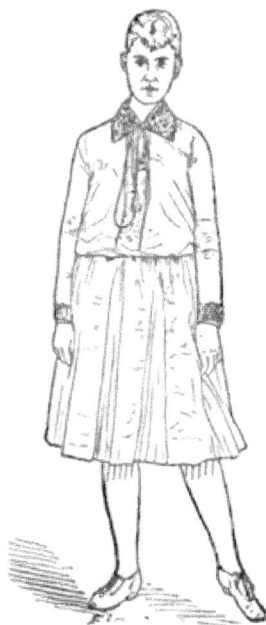

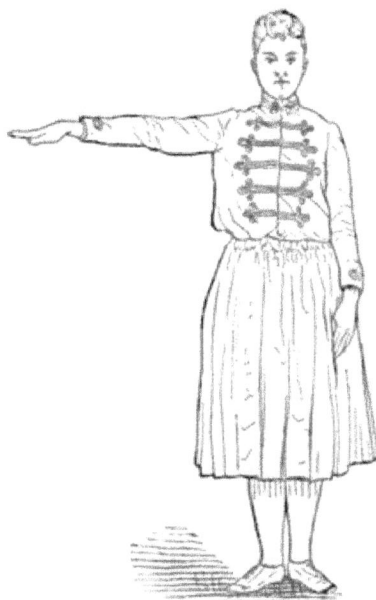

Fig. 38.   Fig. 39.

Fig. 38.—Swinging motion of the leg.
Fig. 39.—Arms shoulder-high to side, **or swinging motion.**

differs from a stepping motion inasmuch as the foot does not touch the floor when out of position. The length of a swinging motion for the leg is about twelve inches, but it can be varied, of course, to suit the wishes of the teacher (Fig. 38).

A swinging motion for the arm is made by swinging

the rigid arm from the side to any of the directions given, or to any desired height (Fig. 39).

8. **Raising and Lowering,** applicable to the arms, legs, and body, is made by raising the knee up to the **front** (Fig. 40), raising the ball of the foot from the floor, while the heel remains on the floor, or by keeping the knees

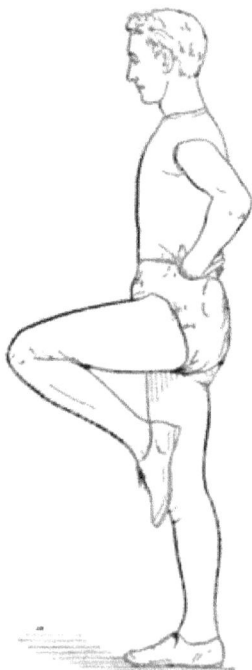

FIG. 40.—Flexing the thigh. FIG. 41.—Flexing the leg.

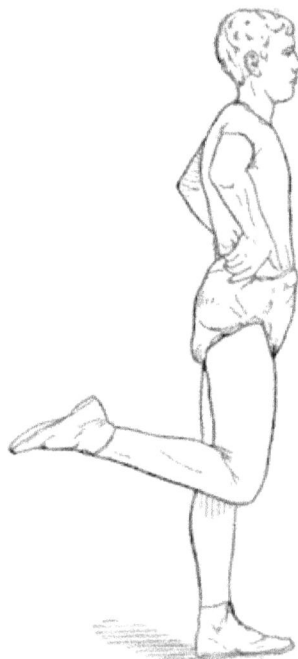

in the same line, raising the heel up and back (Fig. 41). The body is raised by standing on tip-toes.

A lowering motion can be made when an arm has been raised. It can be made forcible, or the arm can drop to the side. The body can be lowered by bendees to the

ing the knees and allowing the body to sink down until the heels touch, or nearly touch, the back of the thigh. In this exercise the trunk is in an upright position; the heels are off the floor (Fig. 42).

9. Twisting **Motions.** — Keep the shoulders to the front, but turn the face to the right or left (Fig. 43). Without moving the feet, turn the shoulders to the right or left. In this case the body turns on the ankles. Keep the heel on the floor and twist the ball of the foot to the right or left, or swing the leg front or to the right, and twist it from left to

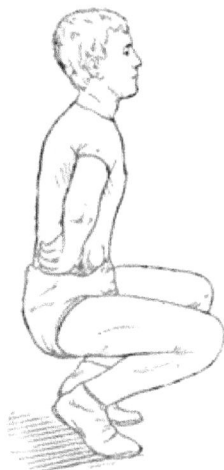

FIG. 42.
Lowering the body.

right. The foot alone cannot be twisted; it can be flexed, extended, or slightly bent. This may also apply to the full-length arm, — it can be twisted to the right or left.

The fore-arm and hand can be twisted, but not the hand alone.

10. Bending Motions, or, as they may be called, flexing motions, apply to the head and neck (Figs. 44 and 45), trunk (Figs. 46 and 47), arms, and legs. They consist in bending the head or trunk in one direction a certain distance, when the bending ceases, and another exercise is necessary to

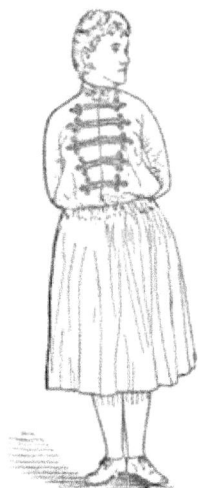

FIG. 43.
Turning the face to the left.

bring the body to its normal position, such as a straightening motion.

The arm can be bent in but one way ; that is, by bringing the hand toward some part of the shoulder.

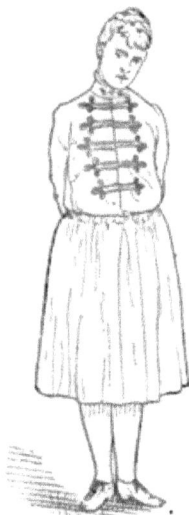

FIG. 44.
Bending the head to the **left.**

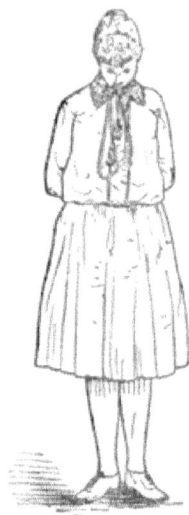

FIG. 45.
Bending the head forward.

The leg can be bent by bringing the heel to the back thigh. The **term " leg "** is applied **to that** part below **the knee.** The part above is **called the** thigh. **The** thigh can be flexed to the front. **These two** bending motions **of** the leg **are** different, **and** bring into **action** separate sets of **muscles.** The hand can be flexed on **the** front **fore-arm.** A straightening is **antagonistic** to **a** flexing motion.

11. Thrusting.—The hands (closed **or** holding some light apparatus) are extended, straightened, or thrust

to one of the given directions. At the finish of a
thrust, the arms are straight. The palms of the
hands may be turned down, front, or up.

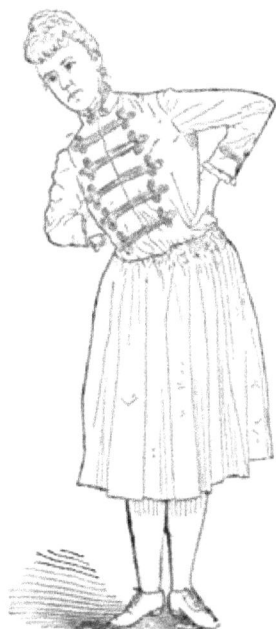

Fig. 46.
Bending body to the right.

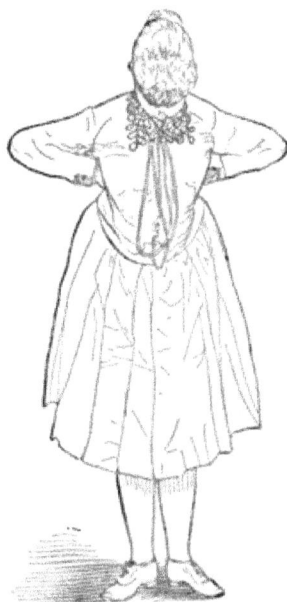

Fig. 47.
Bending the body forward.

12. **Rolling** applies to the head, trunk, and eyes.
The head or trunk is bent in one direction. From this
position it rolls around in a circle, or part of a circle,
from right to left, or left to right. In certain exercises
the eyes are rolled.

13. Opening **and Closing** applies to the hands, eyes,
and mouth. The hands are opened wide, and the
fingers spread apart; to close the hands, clinch the
fist.

The correct **way to** shut **the hand** is seen in Fig. **176.**

The eyes and mouth are opened and **closed in some** grotesque exercises.

14. **Slapping Movement** is made by striking the **hands** together. This exercise can **be** executed with **the** hands down in front **or** back, **the** back exercise **being** especially good, **with the hands** up or front, the **arms** being rigid or with **bent arms** in front, the hands held elbow high. **When teaching** children to keep **time or** to march, the slapping **exercise is** of aid, as it **shows** when the **accent** should **come, and that it** should come with the left foot.

15. **Stamping** Movements are made by raising the foot only two or three inches **from** the floor, and bringing **it** down forcibly, allowing the heel and ball **to** strike the floor. This exercise is useful **for teaching** children to mark time, and **to** teach them the difference between the right and left foot. **In** this case the stamping is only to be done with the **left foot.** The stamping exercise, if made on certain counts, can also be used **to** catch the step when running.

16. **Circling Movements** apply particularly **to** the arms. They are made by swinging the full arm **in** a circle from side to side, or from front to rear. The hand can start from the chest, make this circle, and return **to** the chest, at the finish making what is called a " heart-shaped circle" (see exercises with the clubs; also the second series with the bells, Fig. 114). It is not so easy to make an accurate movement when circling as it is to make an angular movement, but more

muscles are used in this exercise than in simple extension or flexion.

17. **Percussing** is made by striking lightly, with the fingers, some part of the thorax. The motion is rapid, but not of sufficient force to cause any unpleasant results. See full description of percussing, page 78.

18. Shrugging is made by raising one or both shoulders. In this exercise do not bend the body. Move only the shoulder.

19. Breathing Exercises are those which cause the lungs to be well filled and emptied. For a more complete description, see page 194.

CHAPTER V.

THIS arrangement of exercises will be found service-able in teaching pupils the cardinal points and the a, b, c's of light gymnastics. It will assist them in learning the regular series that are to follow, whether they are in free gymnastics, where no apparatus is used, or in light gymnastics, with bells, wands, swords, etc.

Arms—Practice Series.—Position, that of attention; music, march time.

1. Bring the right hand to the hip, the thumb and elbow well back, four times. The same with the left hand four times, and both hands eight times; unless otherwise stated, the counts for exercises in this series will be the same as here given. When using both hands, touch the thumbs back (Fig. 30).

2. Bring the right hand, closed, to the chest; left hand; both hands.

3. Bring the right hand to the shoulder; left hand; both hands (Fig. 29).

4. Swing the right arm, rigid, shoulder-high, to the right (Fig. 39); left arm; both arms; also drill the pupils in swinging the arms in the oblique and front directions, hip-high, head-high, shoulder-high.

5. Swing the right arm, rigid, FRONT and UP; left arm; both arms.

70

6. Bring the right hand, palm down, to the left shoulder; bring the left hand to the right shoulder; both.

7. Fold the arms in front 8 times (Fig. 31).

8. Fold the arms back 8 times (Fig. 32).

9. Swing the arms up sideways and clasp the hands back of the head (keep the elbows back) 8 times.

10. Flex the arms forcibly, palms of the hands front, elbows back (Fig. 48).

Legs and Feet.—1. Keep the toes on the floor, but raise the right heel by bending the knee (same with the left), 8 times each.

Do not in this exercise permit the hip to drop.

2. Keep the heel on the floor, raise the toes and twist the right leg to the right or left; same with the left.

3. Flex the right thigh until it is parallel to the floor, point the toes down; same with left (Fig. 40).

4. Flex the right leg, keeping the thighs parallel to each other. Point the toes back. Same with the left (Fig. 41).

5. Swing the right leg in the directions given, 8 times each. Same with the left (Fig. 38).

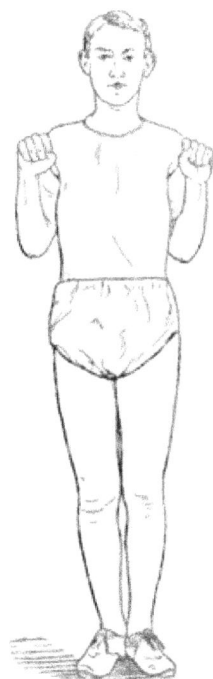

FIG. 48.
Flexing the arms,
palms front.

6. Take the hopping motions on each leg, both legs, and alternate. The alternate motion can be easily turned to a " run in place " (Fig. 37).

7. The stamping motion with the right foot ; **same**
with the left.

Body.—1.   Bend the body forward to each side, and
back **also, in** the oblique directions, 8 times each (Figs.
46 and **47**).

2. **Turn** the shoulders to the right **and** left, **8** times
each.

3. Roll **the body from left to right,** and right **to**
left, 8 times.

4. Take **the same exercises with** the head that **are**
given for the **trunk.** In some cases pupils should **be**
excused from **the head motions, as they** become dizzy.

CHAPTER VI.

THE following four series in free gymnastics will be found serviceable.

The following simple exercises can be given in the school-room :

FIRST SERIES.

March Time.

Position, that of a soldier, but hands on the hips, thumbs forward.

1. Raise on the toes 16 times.
2. Raise on the heels 16 times.
3. Bend the body forward 8 times (Fig 47).
4. Bend the body right side 8 times (Fig. 46).
5. Bend the body left side 8 times.
6. Bend the body back 8 times.
7. Drop the head to right side 12 times.
8. Drop the head to left side 12 times.
9. Drop the head back 8 times; at same time bring hands to chest (Fig. 32).
10. Thrust clinched hands down 8 times.
11. Thrust clinched hands out 8 times.
12. Thrust hands up 8 times.

73

13. Thrust hands front 8 times, and drop them at the side on the eighth count.

14. Bend right knee (keep toes on floor) 8 times.

15. Bend left knee (keep toes on floor) 8 times. On the fourth count, flex the arms, elbows at the side, palms front, hands open, fingers apart.

16. Open and close hands 16 times. On the sixteenth count, let hands fall at the side.

17. Stamp the left foot lightly 16 times.

18. Stamp the left foot and slap the hands 16 times.

19. Stamp the left foot, slap the hands, and count out loud 16 times.

The exercises 17, 18, 19 are for small children, and are used especially to teach them to keep time and to mark time.

SECOND SERIES.

Waltz Time, 8 *counts to each movement.*

Position, that of a soldier, but hands resting naturally at side.

1. Step right foot diagonally forward to the right (Fig. 33).

2. Same with left foot.

3. Right foot diagonally back.

4. Same with left foot.

5. Step right foot over in front of left, touch toes to floor, and bring back.

6. Same with left.

7. Swing the right arm sidewise above and slightly over the head, palm down, arm curved.

8. Same with the left.

9. With both. As the hands come down on the last count, clasp them below in front, backs of the hands up.

10. Step right foot diagonally back and across the left, touch only the toes to the floor, incline the body slightly forward (bowing motions).

11. Same with left.

12. Swing the clasped hands above the head and step right foot across in front of the left; incline the body slightly to right.

13. Same with the left.

THIRD SERIES.

March Time, each movement 8 times.

Position, same as that of a soldier, except that the hands rest on the hips, fingers back.

1. Raise right foot back, keep knees together (Fig. 41).

2. Same with the left.

3. Raise right knee front, toes pointing down, bending leg, body erect.

4. Same with left (Fig. 40).

5. Swing right leg (rigid) to right side.

6. Same with left (Fig. 38).

7. Twist shoulders to right; do not bend legs or raise feet.

8. Same to left.

9. Turn head to the right.

10. Same to left (Fig. 29).

11. Drop head back, hands at side on the eighth count.

12. Force the head back, trying to touch the chin to the throat.

13. Shrug the right shoulder **on** count one; on count **two,** raise right arm (rigid), shoulder-high, to side, and lower it; on count three, shrug shoulder; on count four, raise the arm again; and so on through 16 counts.

14. Same with left arm.

15. Same with both arms.

16. Raise right arm (rigid) shoulder-high to the front, swing smartly to the right side, shoulder-high, back to front, down at the side, palm up. This movement takes four counts. Repeat to 16 counts.

17. Same with the left.

18. Raise both arms to the front, swing to side, shoulder-high; and on counts three and four, slap the hands together smartly back of the body below the waist. Take this for 16 counts.

FOURTH SERIES.

March Time.

Position, that of a soldier. The following movements are arranged from *Upton's Tactics,* and are well adapted for drawing the shoulders back and producing an upright carriage of the body. They have been arranged for music. Each exercise, 16 or 32 counts.

First Exercise.

Count 1, swing the arms sideways and up (the hands can be slapped in this movement). 2. Force the arms to the position seen in Fig. 48. Thrust the arms back to position No. 1. 4. Force the arms obliquely back and down.

Second Exercise.

1. Raise the arms from the sides, extend to their full length till the hands meet above the head, palms of the hands to the front, fingers pointing upward, thumbs locked, right thumb in front, the shoulders pressed back. 2. Bend over till the hands, if possible, touch the ground, keeping the arms and knees straight. 3. Come to position of No. 1. 4. Hands at the side.

Third Exercise.

1. Extend the arms horizontally to the front, the palms of the hands touching. 2. Throw the arms extended well to the rear, inclining slightly downward, at the same time raise the body upon the toes. 3. Come to position as No. 1. 4. Resume the position of the soldier.

The first and second motions of this exercise can be continued by the commands *one, two, one, two*, till the seventh count. With practice, scholars will be able to touch the hands behind the back.

Fourth Exercise.

On count 1, raise both arms, rigid, shoulder to the side, palms up. 2 and 3. Make short circles from front to rear with the arms. This part has been called " grinding the shoulders." 4. Force the hands down to the side. Palms front. Do not let the hands bound away from the thighs.

PERCUSSING MOVEMENTS.

These exercises are a part of the manipulation movements. They tend to increase the circulation,

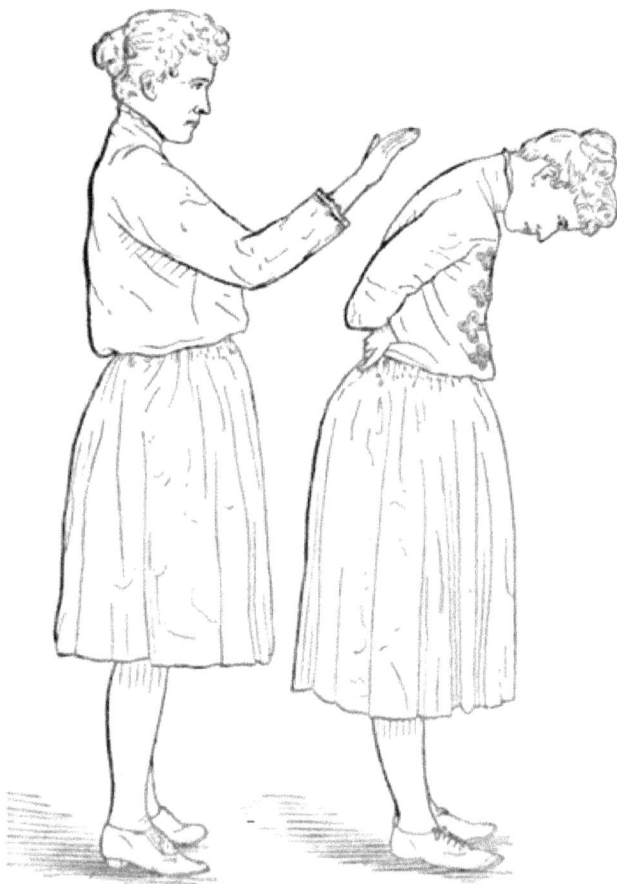

Fig. 49.—Position for percussing the back.

change tissue, and force the air to all parts of the lungs. They are as good for adults as for children. All striking movements are executed rapidly, to polka or galop time ; the beat being made on some part of the thorax with the ends of the fingers, not with the flat hand or fist.

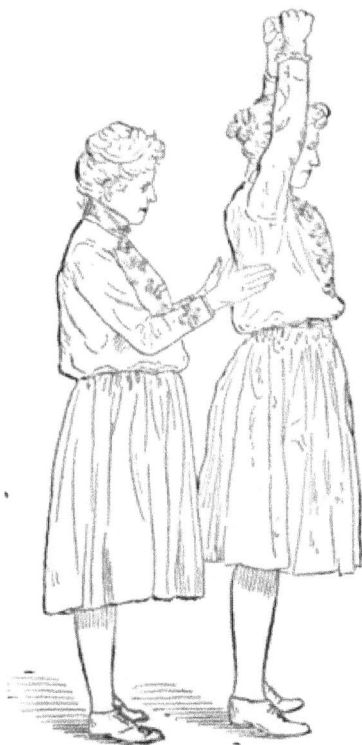 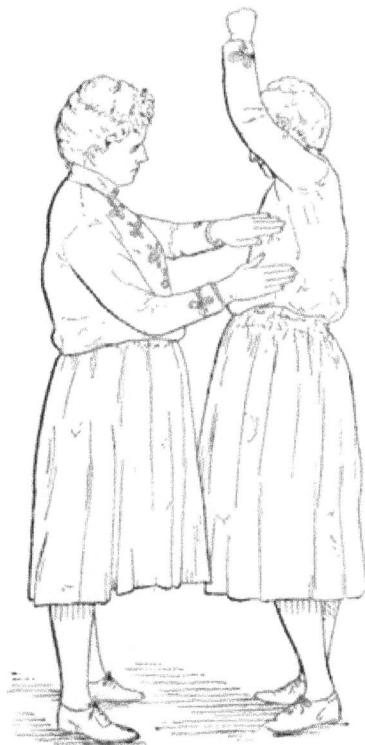

FIG. 50.   FIG. 50a.

Positions for percussing the side.

1st Exercise. Teach pupils to percuss their own chests until they have a definite idea of how the exercise is executed.

2d Exercise.   Form the class in " twos," and com-

mand all to right or left face. This will bring the
pupils so that one stands back of the other. (See Fig.
49.) The pupil in front places the hands on his
hips and bends the body slightly forward, thus pre-
senting the back for percussion. The rear pupil takes
the position seen in Fig. 49. The exercise begins with

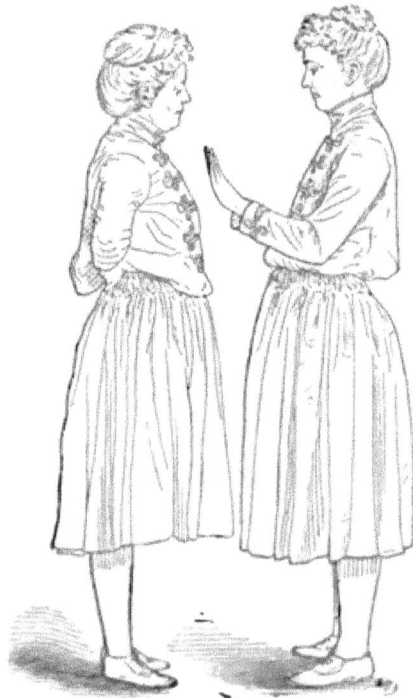

FIG. 51.—Position for percussing the chest.

the music at the command READY! and lasts for 32
counts. At a chord, the class faces about and No. 1
takes the striking exercise.

3d Exercise. At the third chord, the pupils again
face about and take the position seen in Fig. 50.

No. 1 curves the arms over the head, thus exposing the sides of the thorax for percussion. The change is made at the chord. This exercise can be lengthened by permitting No. 1 to raise the right arm above the head while No. 2 percusses with both hands on one side (Fig. 50¹).

4th Exercise. The two pupils face each other. No. 2 percusses the chest of No. 1, who at the chord takes the exercise. At another chord, both pupils raise the hands and percuss the chest of their neighbor. This exercise can be varied by forming a file of pupils and allowing them to beat the backs or sides of those in front of them, and having the pupils about face at a chord, as when formed in twos, to continue the movements. If the file is long, a circle can be formed and the same exercise taken.

The musician plays for 32 counts, stops, strikes a quick chord for facing, and continues with the polka. It is desirable that the music be of a popular character. Pupils can form two's and take their places by chords so that after a few drills the entire exercise can be taken without command.

It will be found amusing as well as beneficial.

CHAPTER VII.

WANDS.

For all exercises given and described under Wands, with the exception of the Manual of Arms and the Bayonet Drill, we use a short stick 30 inches in length and $\frac{5}{8}$ of an inch in diameter. These sticks can be purchased at hardware stores for about one cent each. They are a little over 3 feet in length, but can be easily cut to the desired length. It makes the stick smoother to have it sandpapered; this the school-boys can do. The author uses these sticks, or "dowels," as they are called, almost entirely. They are not only good for the wand exercises, but they can be used for fencing and single-stick, while they are far less expensive than the regular wand.

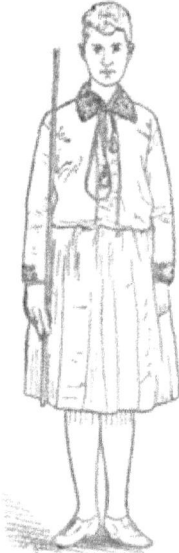

For the Manual of Arms and the Bayonet Drill, use a wand 4 feet 6 inches in length; but otherwise the short stick is better for class work, as it does not require the space for exercising that the longer ones do. Again, the dowels can be cut to fit the width of the desks when they are to

Fig. 52.
Carry arms.

82

be used in the class-room, so that each pupil can
take care of his own wand. For gymnasium use, the
wands may be kept in a box 18 inches square and 2
feet high ; or a box attached to the side of the house
may be used. Racks are
not satisfactory, as too much
time is required to take and
replace the sticks. The following are the A, B, C, or
the preliminary exercises, for
the wands. It is necessary
that the teacher should thoroughly understand them before he attempts to teach
them to a class :

I. CARRY ARMS. (See Fig.
52.) This should be the position of the wand when it is
taken from the box or when
the class is marching. The
wand is held by the thumb
and first two fingers.

II. *Wand* DOWN. Drop the
wand to the position seen in

FIG 53 — Wand down.

Fig. 53 ; the hands are the width of the shoulders
apart ; backs of the hands are front.

III. *Right hand* OUT. (See Fig. 54.) Swing the
wand shoulder-high to the right, the right arm extended in the same direction, the back of the left hand
resting near the base of the neck ; the shoulders are to
the front. The same position is taken on the left.

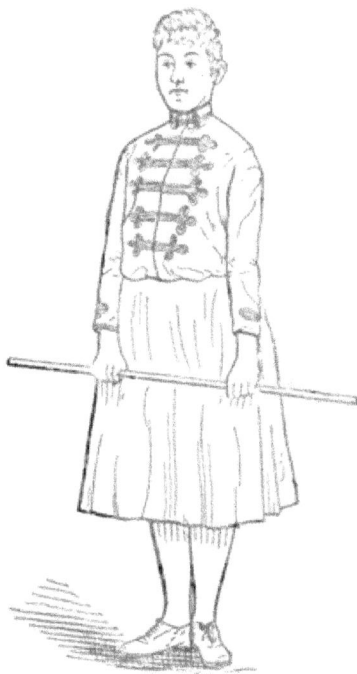

IV. *Wand* UP. Swing the wand to arm's length above the head, wand parallel to the floor. (See Fig. 55.)

V. *Wand* FRONT. Swing the wand shoulder-high to the front at arm's length, wand parallel to the floor (Fig. 56).

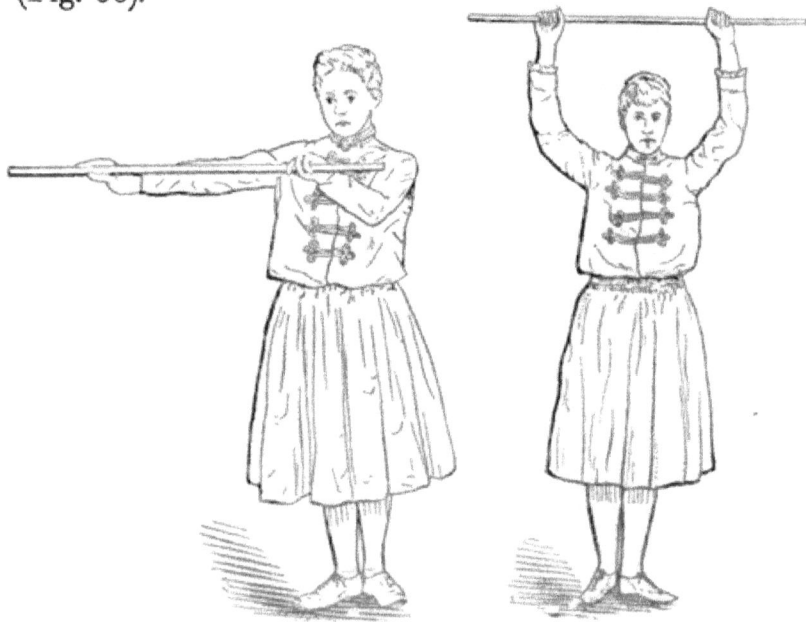

FIG. 54.—Wand out to the right.   FIG. 55.—Wand up.

VI. *Wand* to the CHEST. Bend or flex the arms, bringing the wand to the chest, wand parallel to the floor (Fig. 57). From this position the thrusting motions can be taken, down, up, or front, to the right or left. In a thrusting motion to the right, turn the shoulders in that direction. The wand can also be brought to the chest by flexing the arms and by raising the elbows, shoulder-high, to the side (Fig. 58).

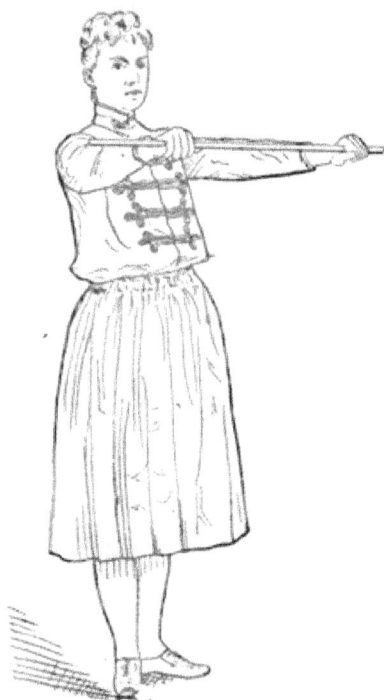

FIG. 56.—Wand front.

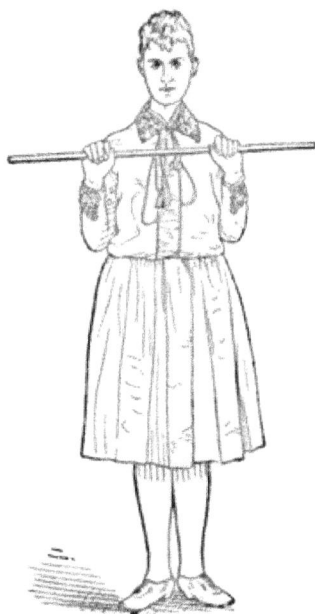

FIG. 57.—Arms flexed.

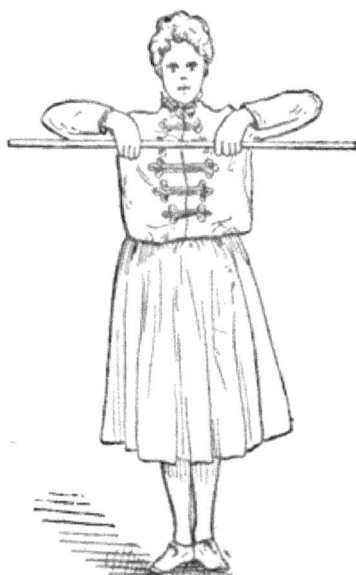

FIG 58.—Elbows shoulder-high to the side.

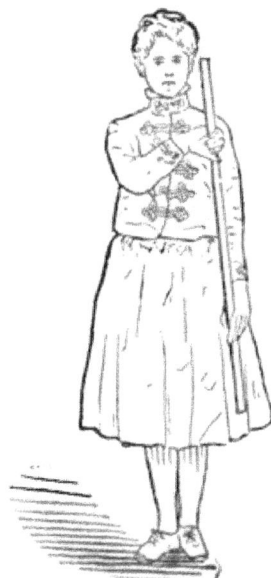

FIG. 59.—Right-hand salute.

VII. *Right-hand* SALUTE. Bring **the** right hand **to the left shoulder, palm of** the **right hand** front; **the left arm** is straight at the side. **A salute** can also **be made** with **the** left **hand.** (See Fig. 59.)

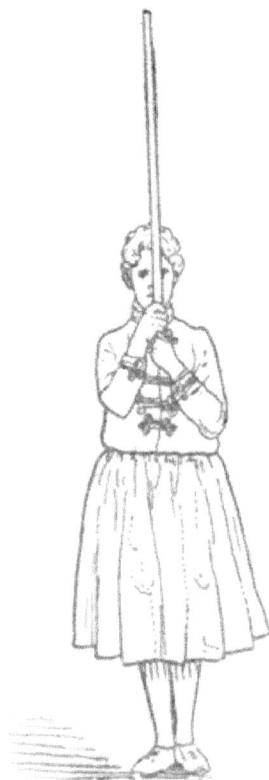

FIG. 60.
Wand in perpendicular position.

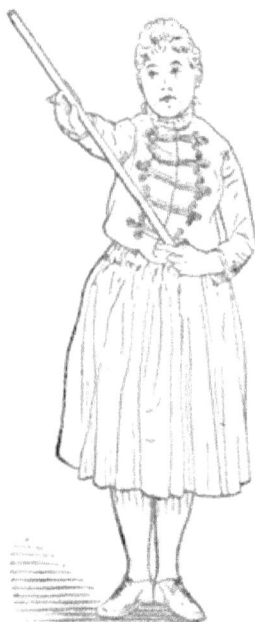

FIG. 61.
Right hand **shoulder-high** diagonally **forward, left** hand waist-high.

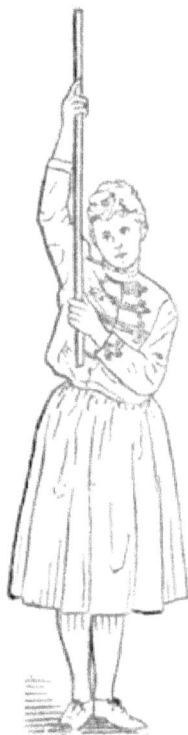

FIG. 62.
Right hand up, **left hand at** right **shoulder.**

VIII. **WAND** TO SHOULDERS, back of **the** head, **wand** parallel **with** the floor (Fig. 67). **If the** wand is **long,** slide the hands to the ends of the wand, **when it may be forced** down **the back** "elbow-high" or to **arm's** length; then, without bending the arms, raise the wands shoulder-high back.

IX. WAND IN A PERPENDICULAR POSITION. Grasp one end of the wand by both hands, the hands the height of the neck. The wand is directly in front of the centre of the face. (See Fig. 60.)

X. RIGHT HAND DIAGONALLY FORWARD to the right, shoulder-high, left hand waist-high in front of the

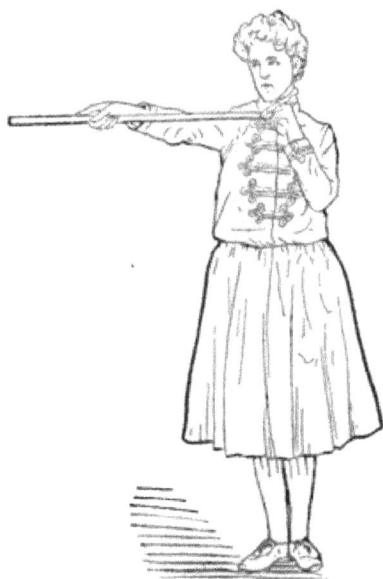 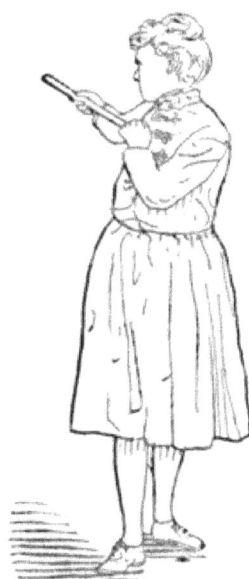

FIG. 63.   FIG. 64.

FIG. 63.—Right hand shoulder-high diagonally forward, left hand at the base of the neck.

FIG. 64.—Right hand points to the rear, left hand at base of the neck.

body. (See Fig. 61.) From the position described in No. III, the right hand may be raised above the head (Fig. 62); it may point to the front or to the back, or in the diagonal directions to the front and back.

These motions, of course, can be taken on both sides. (See Figs. 63, 64, 65.)

XI. "TWISTING MOTIONS." The wand may be held in the center by one hand, and twisted **from right to left.**

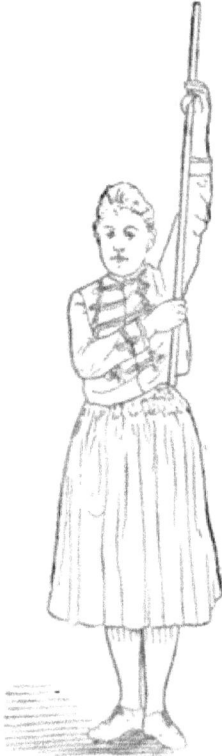

Fig. 65.
Left hand up, right hand
left shoulder.

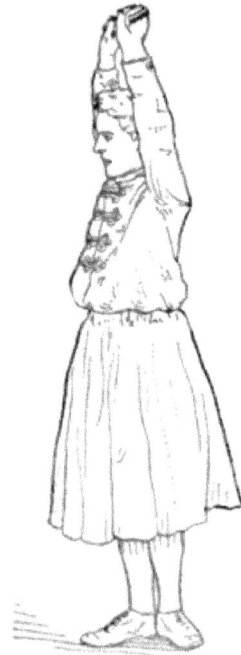

Fig. 66.
Wand up, and twisting motion
to the right.

It may be held FRONT, and turned to a vertical position, right or left hand up.

It may be held UP, and turned so that it points to the

front. This can be done either by the arms alone or by turning the body. (See Fig. 66.)

XII. The motions with the wands given under the head of Preliminary Exercises will either singly or in combination make all the exercises that are described in series 1, 2, and 3; also the marching series.

If they are thoroughly understood, it will be easy to make these combinations.

MARCHING SERIES.

To ordinary march time, the members of the class marching at arm's length from each other, the majority of the preliminary exercises can be executed. It may be necessary to change the time for certain movements, or to take two counts for certain exercises, such as raising the wand up or bringing it to the shoulder.

First Series.   Music, March or Polka Time.

Position, *Wand* at *Carry Arms* (Fig. 52.)

At the chord or count, bring the wand to the first position, or down. (See Fig. 53.)

1. Flex the arms 8 times (Fig. 57).

2. Raise the elbows, shoulder-high, to the side; the wand is brought to the chest 8 times (Fig. 58).

3. Swing the wand, shoulder-high, to the front, arms rigid (Fig. 56).

4. Swing the wand out to the right, parallel to the floor (Fig. 54).

5. The same on the left.

6. Swing the wand up above the head, arms straight (Fig. 55.)

7. Raise the right hand, palm front, to the left shoulder; the left **arm** remains straight at the side (Fig. 59).

8. The same with the left hand.

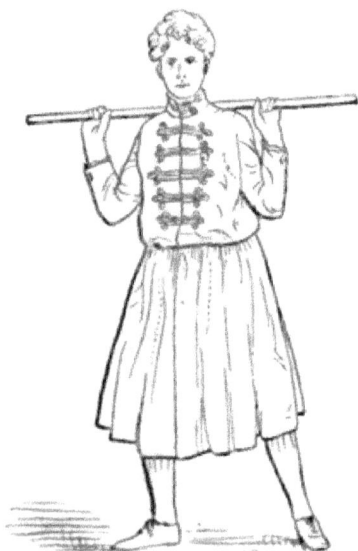

FIG. 67.

Wand on shoulders and **charge to** the right.

9. Swing the right arm, rigid, UP; bring the left hand, palm back, to the right shoulder 8 times (Fig. 62).

10. Swing the left hand up and bring the right hand to the left shoulder (Fig. 65).

11. Raise the right arm, rigid, diagonally forward to the right, shoulder-high. Bring the left hand to the center of the chest and to the base of the neck (Fig. 63).

12. Take the same exercise with the left.

13. Bring the wand to the back of the shoulders, charge the right foot to the right (Fig. 67).

14. Same on left.

15. Swing wand, shoulder-high, front, and step the right foot front 8 times (Fig. 68).

16. Same on the left.

17. Charge right foot diagonally forward, and swing wand up 4 times. Same on left. (See Fig. 69.)

Second Series.   Music, Waltz Time.

Position, same as in **First Series.**

I. Count 1, swing the wand, shoulder high, to the

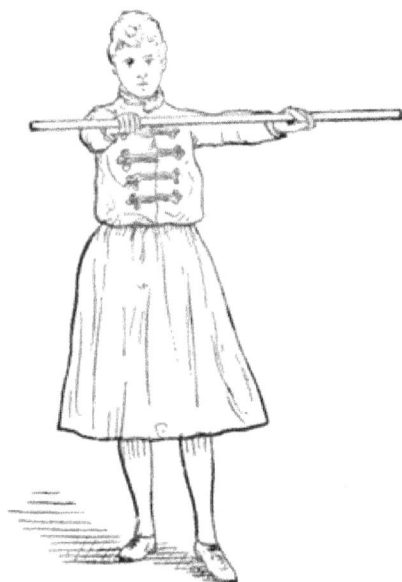

Fig. 68.

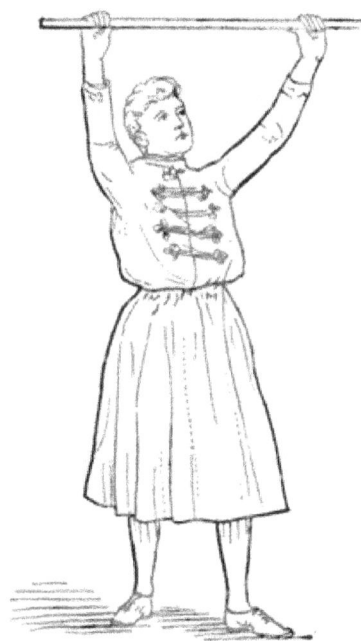

Fig. 69.
Wand up and charging motion with the left foot.

front. From this position, on count 2 swing the wand to the right, and turn the shoulders the same way. Count 3, come back to

position 1, and on count 4 drop the wand to the
position at starting. Take this exercise 16 counts on each side, alternating.

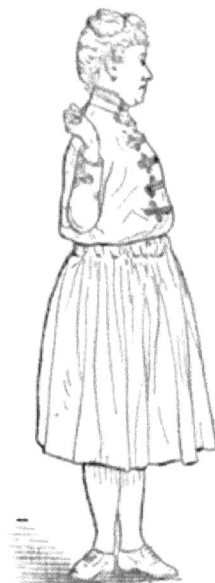

II. Count 1, right face and flex
the arms. Count 2, thrust the wand,
shoulder-high, to the front. Count
3, bring the wand back to the chest.
Count 4, thrust the wand UP. Count
5, bring the wand to the shoulder,
back of the head. Count 6, thrust
the wand UP. Count 7, bring the wand
to the chest. Count 8, come to starting position. At the next count, front
face and take the exercise through
8 counts. Then face to the left and
again front face. This will require
32 counts to finish.

FIG. 70.
**Wand on shoulders
and turn to the left.**

III. Count 1, swing the wand up.
Count 2, twist the wand from right
and left, to front and back ; the right hand front, the
left back, wand parallel to the floor (Fig. 66). Count
3, twist the wand back to position 1. Count 4, wand
down ; take the same exercise but swing the left hand
front on count 2. Full number of counts, 32. On the
last count of 32, bring the wand to the shoulders, back
of head.

IV. Count 1, twist the shoulders to the right and
back, front again. Count 2, same to the left 8 times
(Fig. 70).

V. Count 1, bend the body to the right (Fig. 71); come back to position. Count 2, thrust the wand up. Take the same to the left 8 times.

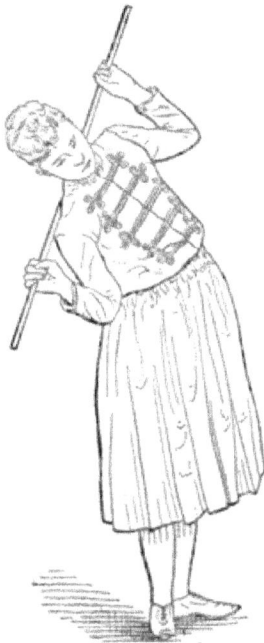

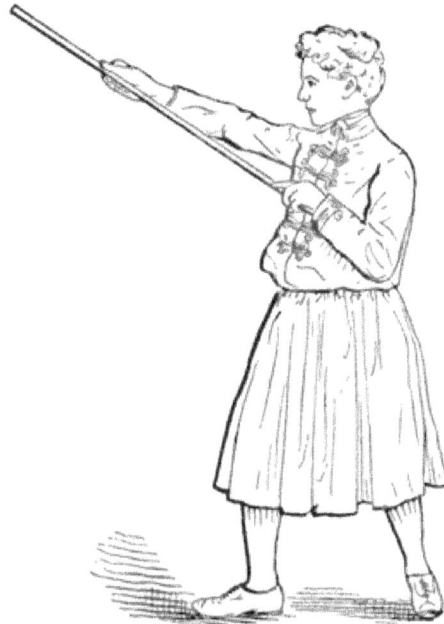

Fig. 71.   Fig. 72.

Fig. 71.—Wand on shoulders and bend to the right.

Fig. 72.—Right hand shoulder-high diagonally forward; right foot charge diagonally forward.

VI. Bring the wand from the shoulders to the chest, and step the right foot diagonally back at the same time. Come back to position and repeat the exercise, but step the left foot diagonally back 8 times. On the 8th count, bring the wand from the shoulder down in front.

VII. Charge the right foot to the right ; the right **arm,** face-high, **to the right;** the left hand **across,** chest-high, **on the** right **(Fig.** 72). Take the charging motion **4 times** to the **right** and 4 times to the left. On the 8th **count,** bring the wand to the position seen in Fig. 60.

VIII. Sliding motion. **The wand is** held **in a perpendicular position in front of the face; the right hand above the left (Fig.** 60) ; charge **the right foot** diagonally **forward to the** right ; slide the **right hand** along **the wand to the** length **of the** arm ; point **the wand** diagonally forward **and** up ; bring **the left hand to the** right shoulder. Fig. 73

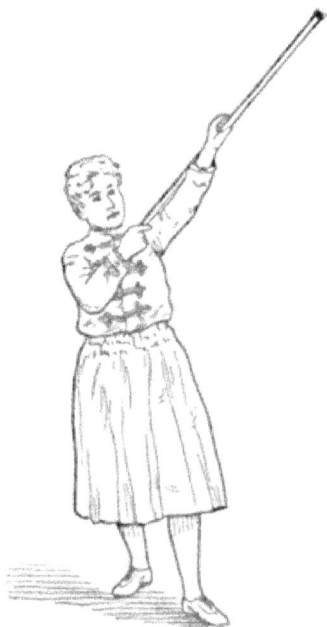

FIG. 73.

Left hand winds diagonally forward and up, right hand chest-**high** in front.

nearly illustrates **this** as **seen** on the left. When coming back **to** position, change hands, the **left above** the right; then **take** this exercise **on the left.** Take this " sliding motion" 8 times, **and** on the **last count** bring the wand DOWN.

IX. Rowing motion. Charge the right foot diagonally forward to the right and raise the wand shoulder-high, front (Fig. 74 illustrates this on the left side), swaying **the** body back, and bring **the** wand to the

chest (Fig. 75). Take the swaying motion 16 counts
on the right. On the last count, wand DOWN; then
take the same on the left.

X. The sixteen-count motion. No. 1, bring the left
hand to the right shoulder. No. 2, raise the right arm,

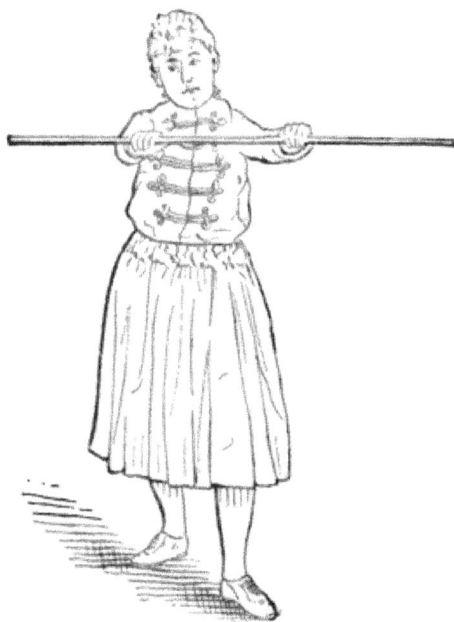

FIG. 74.

First position in rowing motion, body
forward.

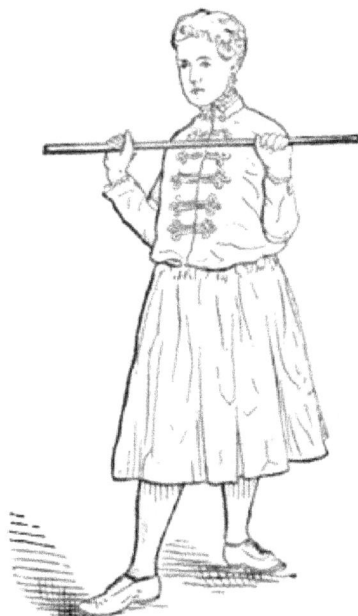

FIG. 75.

Second position in rowing motion,
body sways backward.

shoulder-high, to the right (Fig. 54). No. 3, raise the
right arm up (Fig. 62). No. 4, raise the left arm up (Fig.
55). No. 5, lower the right hand to left shoulder
(Fig. 65). No. 6, lower left arm, shoulder-high, to
the left. No. 7, lower left hand to the side (Fig. 59).

No. 8, wand DOWN. The next 8 counts are just the reverse of the first.

Third Series.   Time, Waltz.

Position, wands down.

Explanatory.—This series is arranged from the German. Every exercise is a four-count movement; that is, it takes 4 counts to finish each exercise. The 4th count always brings the wand back to the starting position, or "wand down." Each exercise is taken two times on a side.

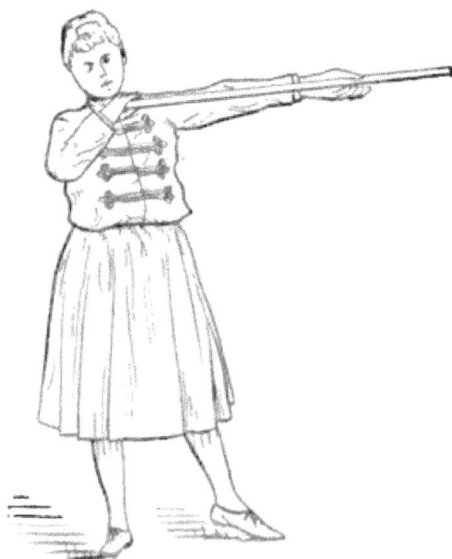 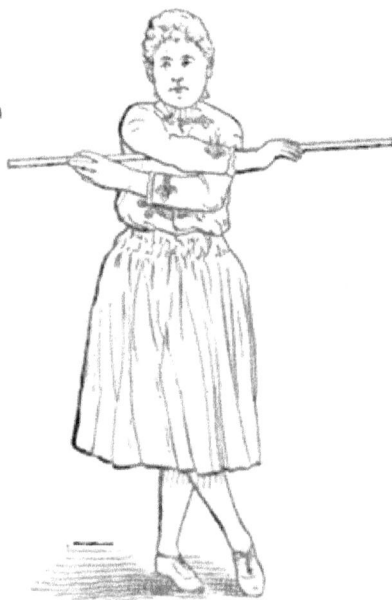

FIG. 76.   FIG. 77.

FIG. 76.—Wand out to the left and stepping motion to the left.

FIG. 77.— Right arm twisted over left, right foot stepping motion **across in front of left.**

I. On **1**, step the right foot to **the right and swing** the **wand out to** the right. **2**, bring the **heels** together and raise **the wand up. 3**, step the **left foot to** the left and lower **wand** out to the left (Fig. 76). **4**, position. Take this, **as** all the following **exercises** are to be taken, **on** the left as well as the right.

II. **1**, charge the right **foot diagonally forward. Raise** the right arm, shoulder-high, **in the** same direction (Fig. 72), left hand waist-high in front, **touching the body. 2**, heels **together, wand** FRONT (Fig. 56). **3**, same as No. **1, but on** the **left side. 4**, position.

III. **1**, charge to the right, **wand** FRONT. **2**, heels together, wand **on shoulder**, back **of neck. 3**, same as No. **1, but on the left side. 4**, position.

IV. **1**, step right foot to the right, wand OUT. **2**, step the right foot over in front of the left, and turn the wand over as seen in **Fig. 77. 3**, come back to position 1. **4**, position.

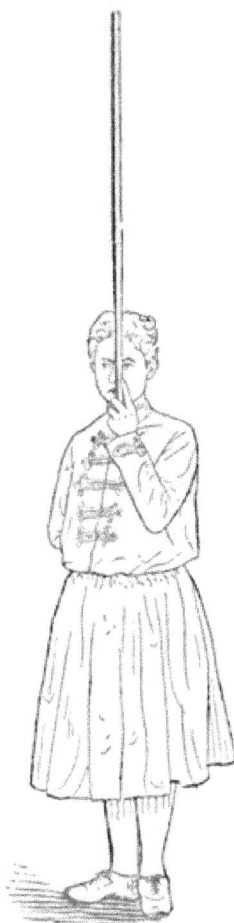

FIG. 78.
Left-hand face salute.

V. **1**, charge the **left foot over** in front of the right ; raise the right arm, shoulder-high, diagonally forward to the right. Fig. 61 shows position of arms. **2**, keep the same position with the

feet, but raise the left hand until the **wand is** FRONT.
Fig. 56 shows position of arms. 3, resume position
No. 1. 4, position.

VI. Charge the right foot diagonally forward to the
right, raise **the** right hand forward, shoulder-high,
left hand **at the** base of the **neck.** Fig. 63 shows
arms. 2, swing the wand to **the** rear, turn the shoulders in the same direction, **but do not** move the feet
(Fig. 64). **3, come back to** position **No. 1. 4, position.**

VII. 1, right oblique face, and bring **the** wand
to the position **seen in Fig. 78. 2,** charge **the** left
foot front and elevate **the
wand. Fig. 169** shows **arm
elevated. 3, come** back to
position No. 1. **4,** position.

VIII. 1, charge the right
foot back and elevate the
right hand back, left hand
across the chest. (See
Fig. 79.) **2, sway** forward
and thrust **the wand forward** and **down, as in Fig.**
109. **3,** come back **to posi-**
tion 1. **4, position.**

IX. 1, left oblique face,
wand **up. 2,** charge the
right **foot** front, bring the left **hand** to the **hip ;**
with the right hand make a circle or mollinet with the
wand to the front, and assume the position in Fig.
3, reverse the circle and come to position in No. 1.

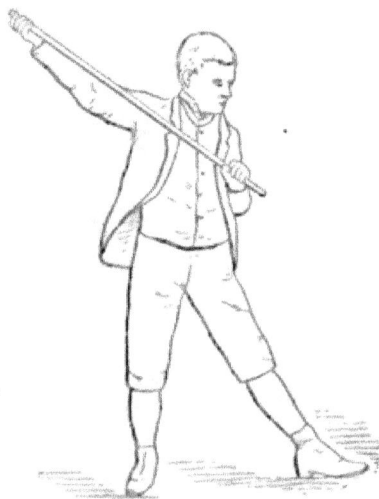

Fig 79.

4, position. (It will be a difficult matter to teach the circle or mollinet to a large class, as the exercise requires skill and practice. The circle is made with the hand and wrist; the wand is grasped very loosely.) The mollinet with the right hand is shown in Fig. 169, page 178.

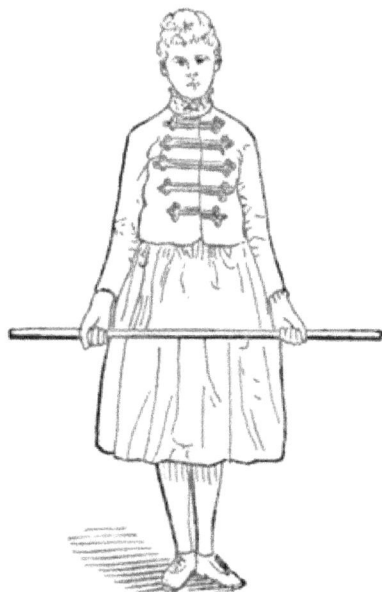 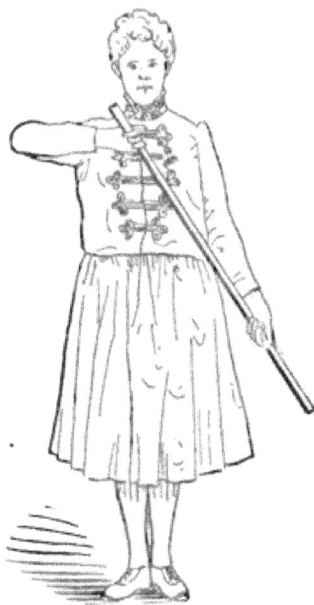

FIG. 80.   FIG. 81.

FIG. 80.—First position of wand for winding motion, palms front.

FIG. 81—Second position of wand for the **winding motion.** (The back of the right hand should be front in this cut.)

Winding Motions.—At the close of No. 4 of exercise IX change the hands so that the palms are front (Fig. 80). Raise the right hand and elbow as in Fig. 81. (In Fig. 81, the back of the right hand is front.) Raise the left hand, shoulder-high, obliquely front, and force the right hand down, as in Fig. 82.

Fig. **83** shows the finish of a winding motion. The winding hand may be held at the side (Fig. **84**), shoulder-high to the front, obliquely front, **or to the side ; as well as** hip-high

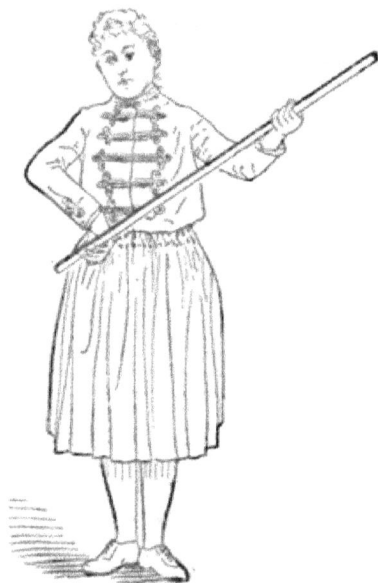

FIG. 82.
Third position of hands in the
winding motion.

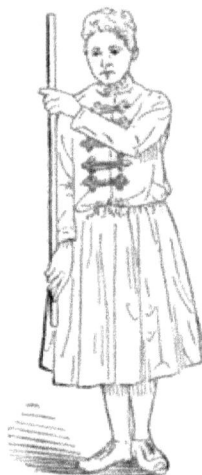

FIG. 83.
Finish of the **winding**
motion

and head-high in either **direction. In the** winding motions keep the hands near the **ends of the** wand. A little practice **will** enable one to wind the wand quickly and easily. These **motions are** at the same time fascinating and puzzling.

X. Charge the right foot diagonally **back** and wind **the** right hand down at the side (Fig. 85). Same on the **left.**

XI. Step the right foot **to the right and** wind the wand out. Same on the left.

XII. Charge the right foot diagonally forward, and wind the wand obliquely forward and up to the right; place the left hand back of the head. Fig. 86 shows arms. Same on the left.

XIII. Charge the right foot front and wind the wand to the position seen in Fig. 83. From this position charge the left foot front and bring the wand chest-

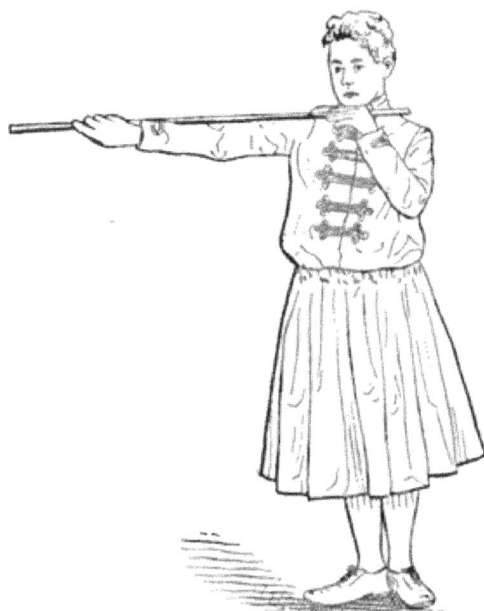 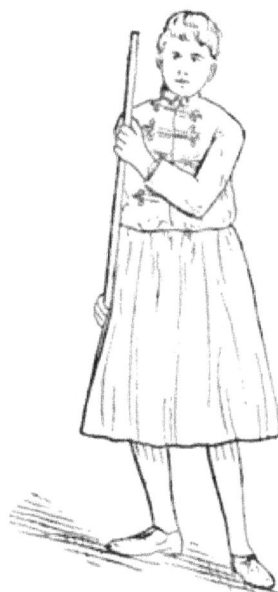

FIG. 84. FIG. 85.

FIG. 84.—Right hand winds shoulder-high to the right, left hand height of the neck.

FIG. 85.—Right hand winds down to the side, left hand shoulder-high on the right; right foot charges diagonally back.

high to the front, palms up. Now wind the left hand out and up to the left, right hand on the chest (Fig. 73). Come from this position back to the first attitude, and from the first attitude to the primary position. **In** this exercise **the** scholar gains ground **by the** second charge.

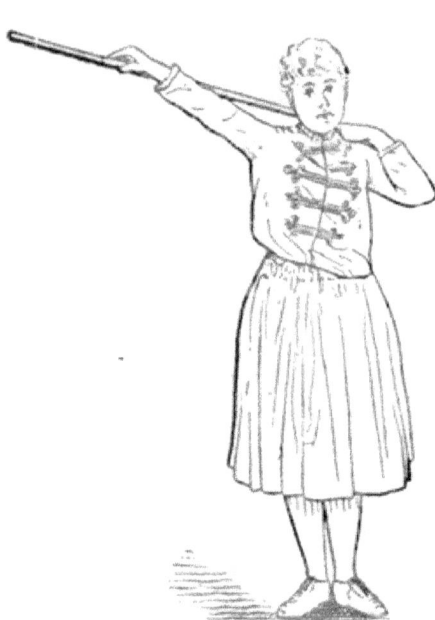

FIG. 86.

Right hand winds **diagonally forward** and up, left hand **back of neck.**

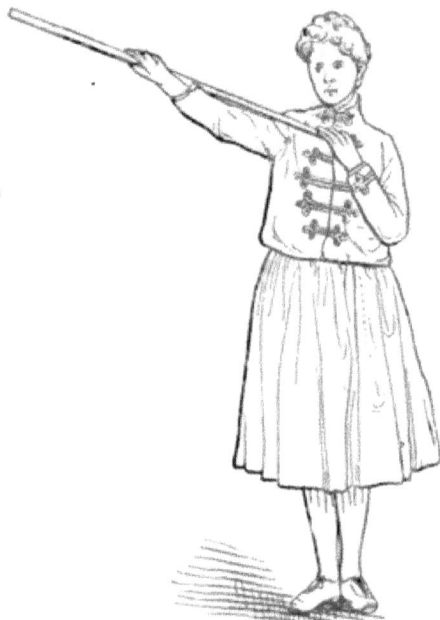

FIG. 87.

Right **hand winds diagonally out and up, left hand chest-high.**

For **all** winding motions, the **waltz** time **is** quickened.

CHAPTER VIII.

MANUAL OF ARMS.

For this exercise, use a wand between four and five feet in length, and about three quarters of an inch in diameter. The movements are executed to march time. It is intended that each motion shall end on four or eight counts. The position is that of " Carry Arms." See Fig. 52.

Present Arms.—Carry the wand to the front and center of the body, the left forearm parallel to the floor, the right arm extended, wand close to the body. Hold this position four counts (Fig. 88).

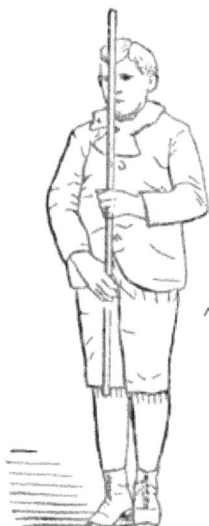

At the command *Carry* ARMS, bring the wand back to the right side, slide the left hand along the wand to the right shoulder, fingers close together, thumb along the first finger, elbow

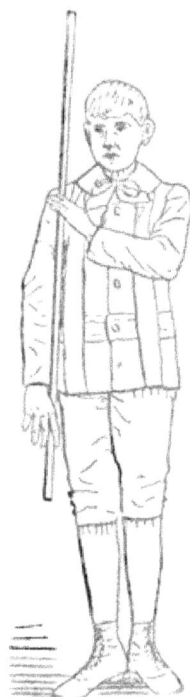

Fig. 88.
Present wands.

Fig. 89.
First position when coming back to carry arms.

103

down ; hold for two counts (Fig. 89).   On 3, drop the left hand to the side.   This exercise **takes** four counts.

Charge Wands.—Execute the first position of *about face*, but step the right foot about **12** inches back of the left ; drop the wand forward until the point is the height of the eye, the right **arm** extended down, the left arm thrown across and in front of the body.   **Grasp** the wand, **as in Fig. 90.   In this** exercise the left **knee**

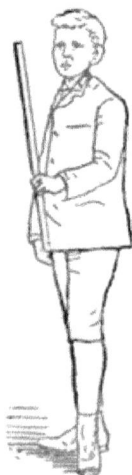

FIG. 90.
Charge bayonets.

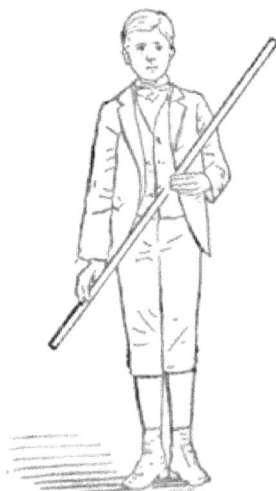

FIG. 91.
Wands port.

is slightly bent, while the weight of the body is thrown a little forward ; hold this position for four counts.

Carry Arms.—In four counts.

Wands Port.—Throw the wand diagonally across the front of the body, and grasp with the left hand, which is elbow-high to the **front** ; the palm of the right hand is above, that of the **left** under, the wand, which is held close to the body. (See Fig. 91.) Four counts.

Carry Wands.—Four counts.

Order Wands.—On Count 1, bring the right hand to the left shoulder, as in Fig. 89 ; but grasp the wand. Count 3, lower the wand quickly to the floor and bring the left hand back to the side.

Parade Rest. — Assume the first position of *about face,*

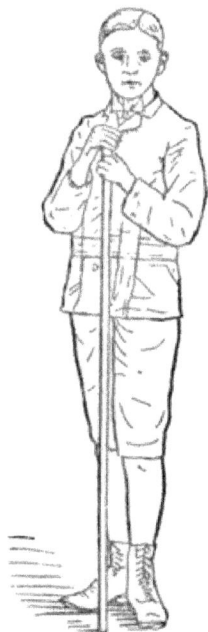

FIG. 92.
Parade rest.

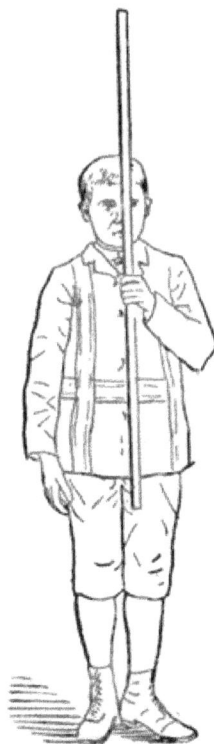

FIG. 93.
Inspect wands.

grasp the wand near the top with the left hand, place the right hand above the left. Four counts. (Fig. 92.) From this position come to ORDER ARMS, four counts.

Carry Wands.—Flex the right arm, at the same time raising the wand and grasping with the left hand just below the right elbow ; the wand is on the right side of the body. This takes two counts. Next, lower the right hand to the side, and raise the left hand, as in Fig. 89. This takes two counts. On 5, lower the left hand to the side, and hold this position through 8 counts.

Inspect Wands.—On Counts 1 and 2, come to *present* WANDS ; on 3, drop the right hand to the side, retain the grasp with the left hand, which is raised very nearly to the height of the chin ; the wand is in front of the center of the body. Hold this position through 8 counts (Fig. 93).

Carry Wands.—Four counts.

Fire.—At Count 1, assume the first position of *about face* ; at the same time drop the wand forward until the end is about the height of the head ; the right hand is elbow-high to the front ; the left hand is chest-high to the front, but on the right side (Fig. 94). On 3 and 4, bring the lower end of the wand to the shoulder, incline the head to the right, and lock along the wand ; the right elbow is nearly shoul-

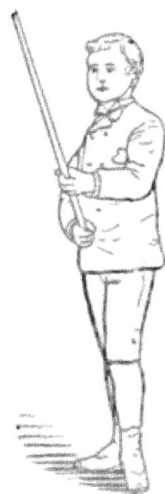

FIG. 94.
First position for firing.

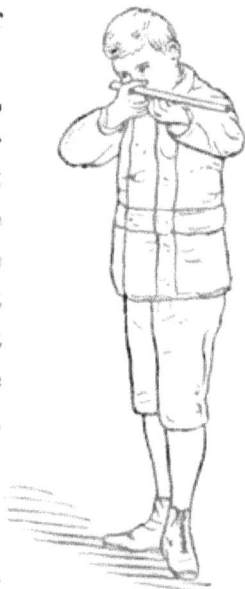

FIG. 95.—Fire.

der-high to the right, the left hand is shoulder-high
to the front on the right side (see Fig. 95); on 5,

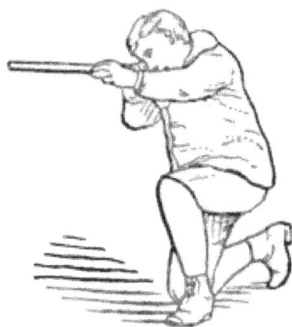

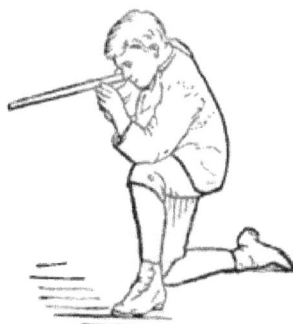

FIG. 96.   FIG. 97.
Two methods of kneeling and firing.

stamp the right foot lightly. Hold this position
through 8 counts.

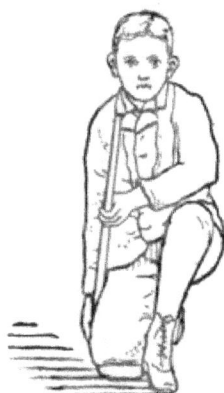

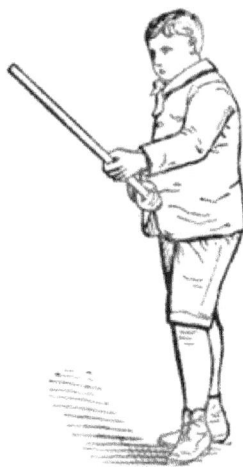

FIG. 98.   FIG. 99.
Kneeling charge.   On guard.

Carry Wands.—Through four counts.
By referring to Upton's Military Tactics, other ex-

ercises can be easily adopted from the Manual of Arms, such as SHOULDER, REVERSE, SECURE, TRAIL. etc.

Figs. 96 and 97 show the method of firing while kneeling ; also a kneeling *charge wands* (Fig. 98).

BAYONET DRILL.

This exercise is taken with the same length wand as the Manual of Arms ; march time ; position the same as that of *charge wands*, but the wand is held more in_ front of the body, the right arm being slightly bent. (See Fig. 99.) This is called " on guard."

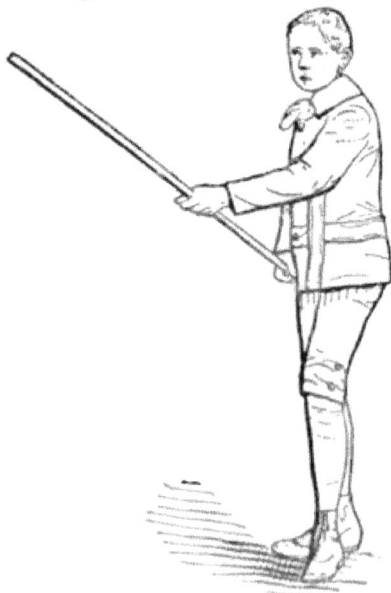

FIG. 100.
Right parry.

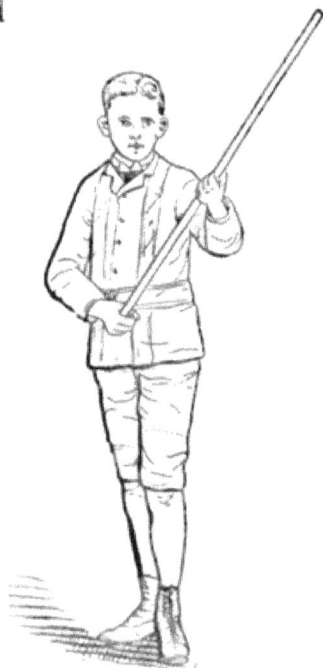

FIG. 101.
Left parry.

Right Parry.—Swing the point of the wand a little to the right. (See Fig. 100.) Hold four counts.

Left Parry.—Swing the point of the wand 6 or 8 inches to the left ; hold 4 counts. (See Fig. 101.)

Right Guard.—Bring the wand to a perpendicular position on the right side 8 inches to the front and the right of the body ; left hand shoulder-high to the right, right hand extended down. (See Fig. 102.)

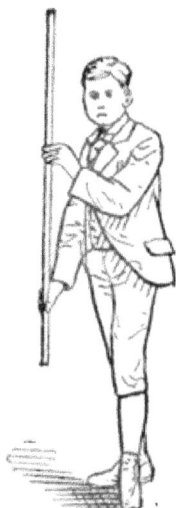

FIG. 102.
Right guard.

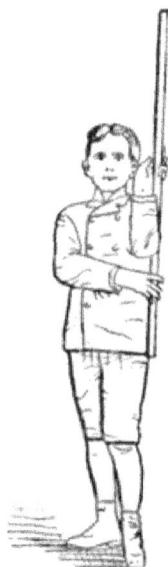

FIG. 103.
Left guard.

Left Guard.—Bring the wand to a corresponding position on the left side, the right hand on the left side a little higher than the hip, the left elbow inside the wand. (See Fig. 103.) Hold 4 counts.

High Guard.—Raise the wand arm's length above the head, parallel to the floor, as in Fig. 104, but keep feet apart.

From the position of *high guard* come to *on guard*. Hold 4 counts.

Thrust to the Rear.—Turn on both heels until the right foot points to the rear, the left foot pointing to the right ; **bring right hand to the chest, left** hand extended to the **front, wand parallel**

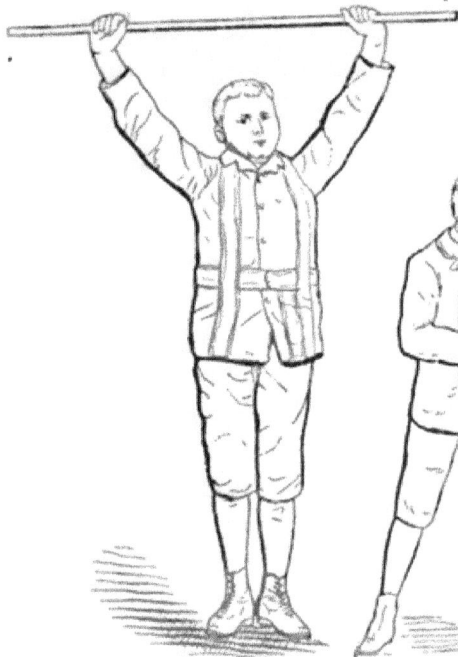

Fɪɢ. 104.—High **guard.**   Fɪɢ. 105.

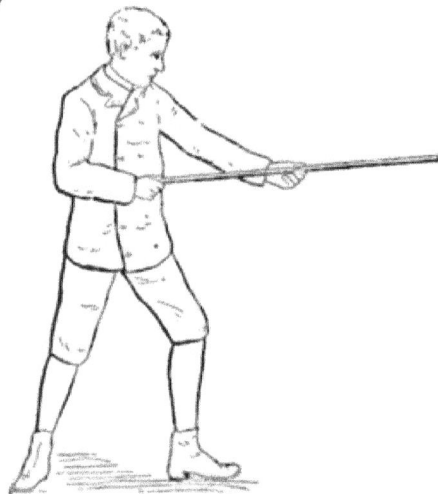

to the floor, face to the rear. Hold four counts. Sway body to the rear, and thrust wand in that direction, wand parallel to the floor. Hold 4 counts. From this position come to *on guard.*

High Thrust.—Sway the body back, thrust right hand back and down, left hand hip-high on the right. (See Fig. 106.) Sway body forward, thrust left hand forward and up, right hand chest-high to the front. (See Fig. 107.)

Middle Thrust.—Sway body back, right arm back, left

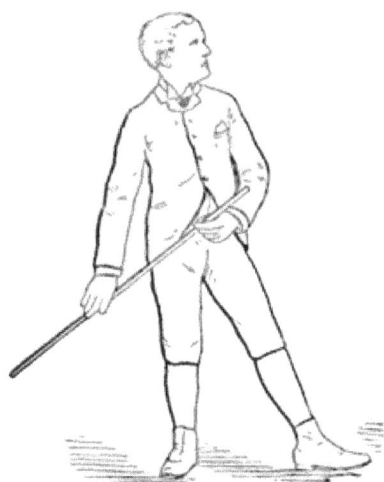

FIG. 106.

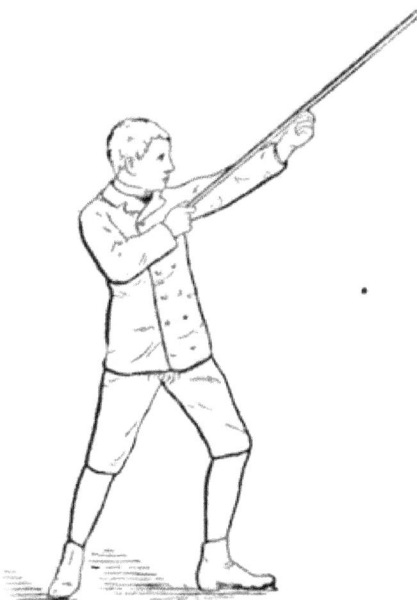

FIG. 107.

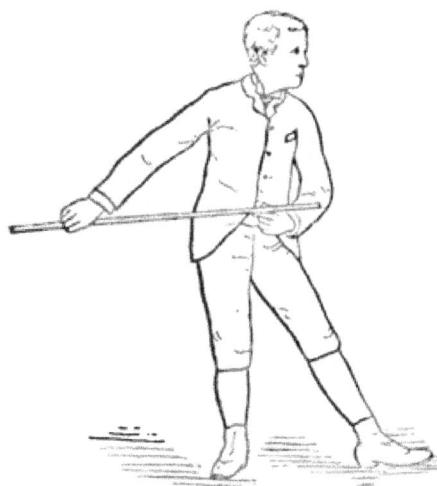

FIG. 108.

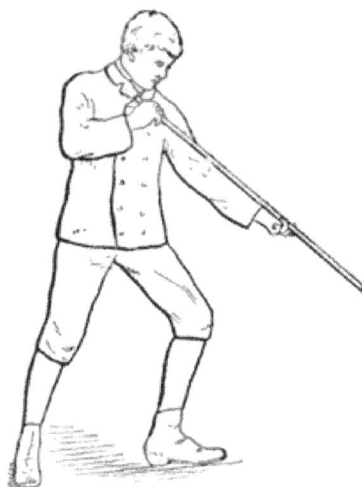

FIG. 109.

hand waist-high on the right side.   The wand is waist-high and parallel to the floor ; 4 counts (Fig. 108). Sway forward, thrust wand forward, as in Fig. 105 ; 4 counts.

Fig. 105 is the finish of a Middle Thrust.   From this position the wand is raised shoulder-high, the

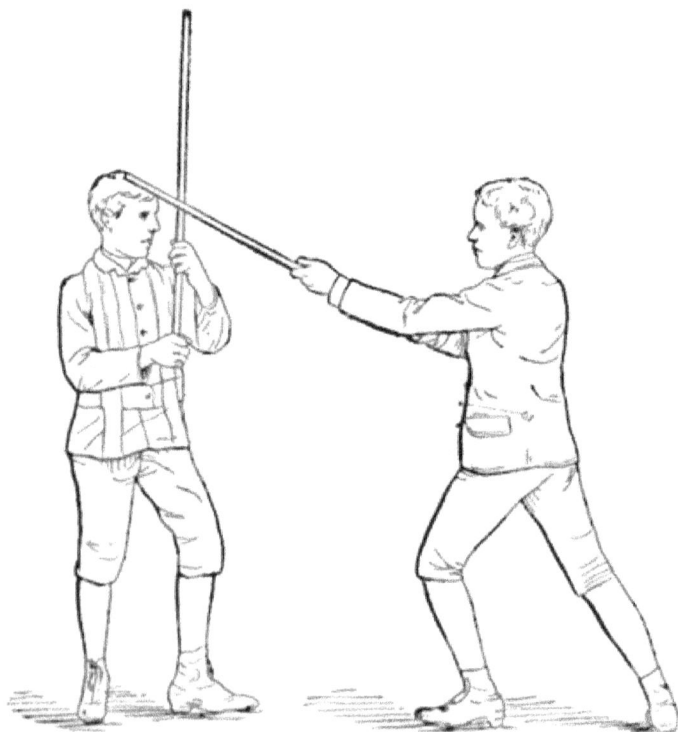

FIG. 110.

face turned back, **and the** rules for Thrust **to the Rear** are followed.

Low Thrust.—Sway body back, right hand back and up, **left** hand chest-high on the right (Fig. 79) ; 4 counts.

Sway body forward, thrust wand forward and down, as in Fig. 109 ; 4 counts. On last count come to position of *carry arms.*

Double Work.—Form the scholars in twos, arranging so that pupils about the same height can work together. The wands are at *carry arms.*

At a chord or at a command, the scholars step apart, face each other, and assume the position of *on*

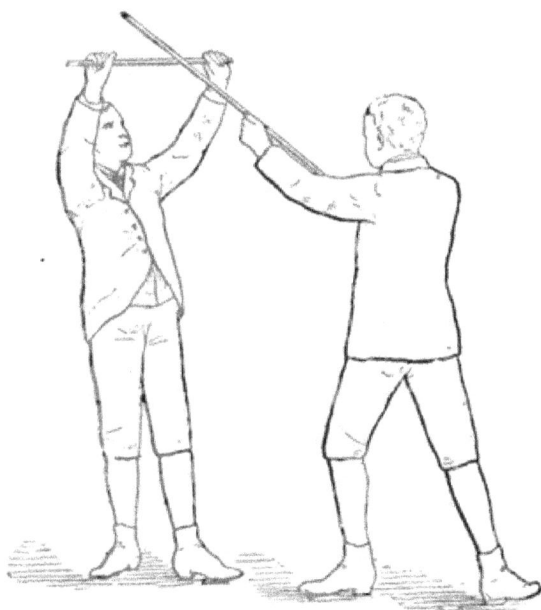

Fig. 111.

guard. The scholar on the right will sway forward and strike lightly with the wand at the right side of his opponent's head, who will assume the position of right guard, which is held for 8 counts. From this position the one on the left will sway forward,

and the one on the right will guard. (See Fig. 110.)
In the same manner take the stroke on the left side
of the head and use the left guard ; also the high
guard. (See Fig. 111.) These positions are merely
postures, and are held for 8 or 16 counts each.

EASY POSTURES FOR WANDS.

Pupils are formed in three rows which are about 5
feet from each other. Arrange the pupils so that
those in front are shortest.

At a chord or command, the first row takes a kneeling charge ;

The second row a *Charge bayonets !*

The third row a FIRE !

This position is held for 16 or 32 counts, when the
scholars will, without a command, assume the second
posture.

First row leans forward, rests the left hand, which
holds the wand, on the floor, turns the face back and
up, raises the right arm back and up, as if warding
off a blow.

The second row takes the first position of a low
thrust, with this exception : the body is swayed forward.

The third row takes a high guard.

These simple attitudes can be given at the end of the
bayonet drill. If more than three rows are exercising,
two rows can take one position. A variety in these
postures can be had if circles instead of rows are

formed and all of the scholars face out. The tallest pupils should stand in the center of the circle. This position is preferable if the pupils are to exercise in the center of the room.

CHAPTER IX.

DUMB-BELLS.

For the weight and method of arranging dumb-bells, see pages 27 and 28.

The series with the bells that are to be described

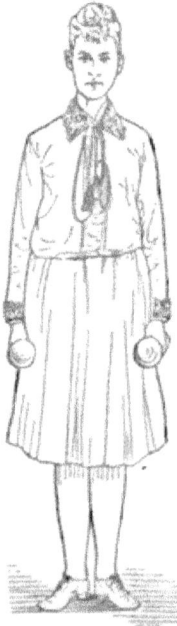

FIG. 112.
First position of the dumb-bells.

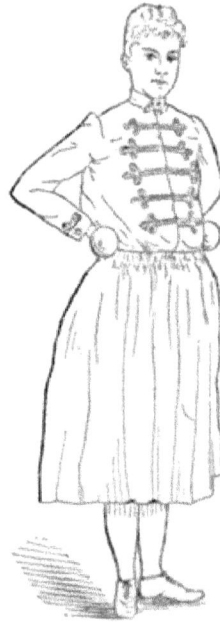

FIG. 113.
Bells on the hips.

in this chapter will be more easily understood if the preliminary motions are well learned. Here, as in Free

Gymnastics and with the Wands, the work is arranged
and should be taught on the principle of A, B, C's.

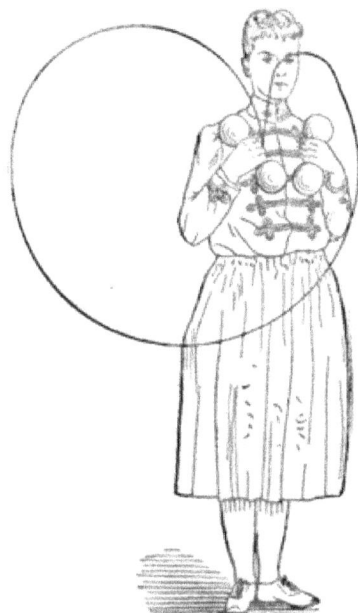

FIG. 114.   FIG. 115.

FIG. 114.—Bells on the chest. The line represents a heart-shaped circle made
with the right hand.
FIG. 115.—Bells on shoulders.

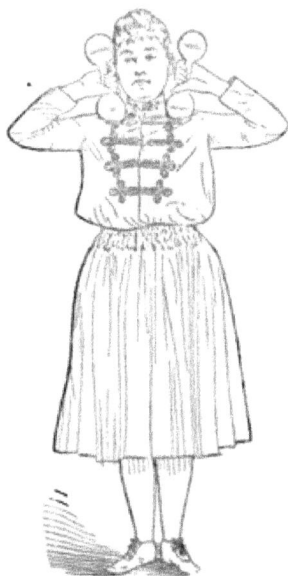

The First Position of dumb-bells: the arms hang
naturally at the side (Fig. 112).

Bells on the Hips.—Same as when the hands are
placed on the hips, the thumb ends front, elbows back
(Fig. 113).

Bells on the Chest No. 1.—The arms are flexed, the
bells form an angle of about 60 degrees, little-finger
ends down (Fig. 114).

Bells on the Chest No. 2.—The thumb ends of the bells

rest against the chest, the little-finger ends point out and slightly up.

Bells on the Shoulders No. 1.—In this case, the palms of the hands are down, elbows shoulder-high to the right. (See left bell and in Fig. 131.)

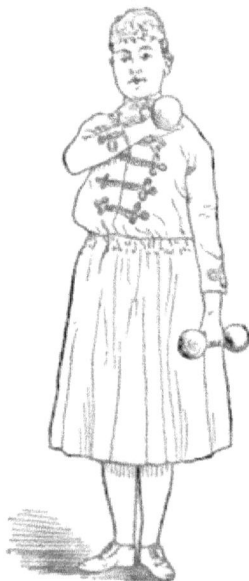

FIG. 116.
Right-hand salute.

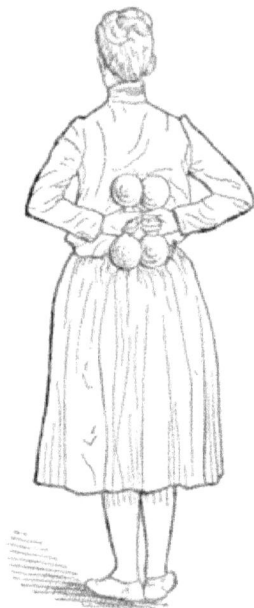

FIG. 117.
Bells at back.

Bells on Shoulders No. 2.—Palms of the hands front, thumb ends down, little-finger ends up. (See Fig. 115.)

Right-hand Salute.—The thumb end of the right bell is brought to the left shoulder, the little-finger end points out and up. This salute is also made with the left hand (Fig. 116).

Bells at the Back—(See Fig. 117.)

Arms Folded in Front—(See Fig. 118.)

Bells Under the Shoulders.—See right bell in Fig. 130.

A Right-angle Motion.—(See Fig. 119.) These positions can be varied by thrusting one hand down and one hand front, or one hand front and one hand up, etc.

With the bells on the chest, they can be thrust DOWN, OUT, UP, or FRONT. They can also be thrust in any of the oblique directions head-high, shoulder-high, and hip-high.

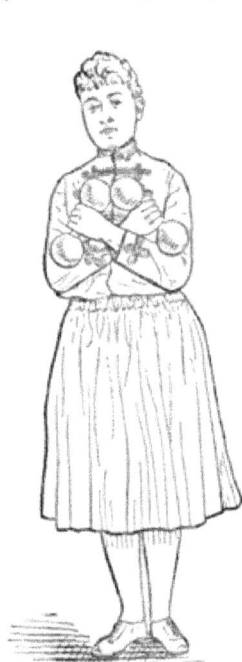

FIG. 118.
Arms folded in front.

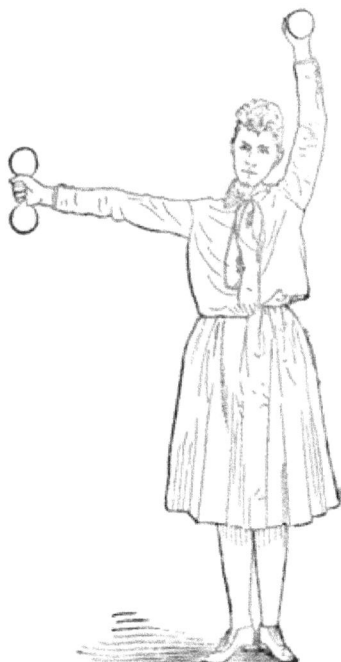

FIG. 119.
Right-angle motion.

A Circling Motion (Fig. 114, R. hand).—This is made on the same principle as heart-shaped circle of the club, which is described on page 140. These circles are made to the right or to the left, with one or both hands.

In executing them, use only the arms.

Flexing Motions and **Swinging Motions** are described under these movements on pages 63 and 65.

Twisting Motions.—The palms of the hands are front, the arms are straight, bells at the side. (See Fig. 120.) The hand is turned so that the thumb points in, while the back of the hand is front. The arm is twisted from the shoulder. (See Fig. 121.)

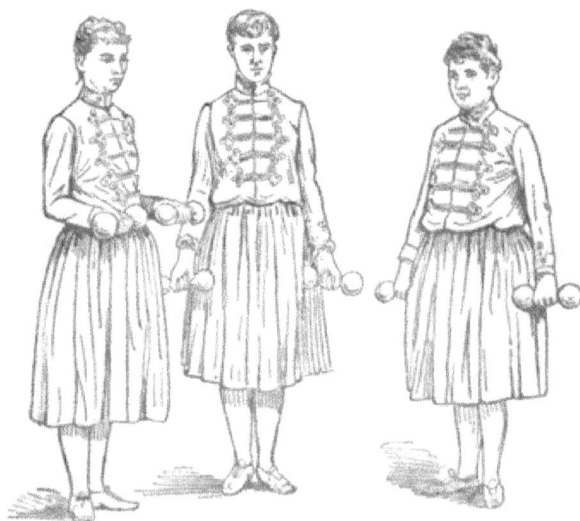

FIG. 122.   FIG. 120.   FIG 121.

FIG. 120.—First position of the bells for twisting motions.

FIG. 121.—Second position of the bells for twisting motion. Notice that the backs of the hands are front.

FIG. 122 shows position for a twisting fore arm motion.

The twisting motions can be taken with the arms OUT, UP, or FRONT. A fore-arm motion can be had if the arms are held as seen in Fig. 122.

The Striking Motions.—The bells may be struck forcibly above the head, the arms swinging up from below, as seen in Fig. 123.   With the arms kept in this posi-

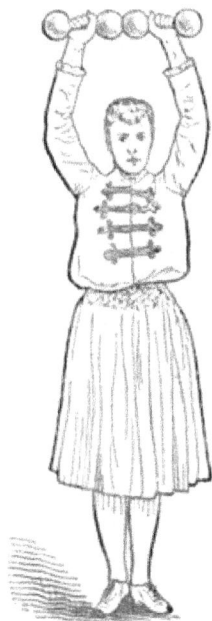

FIG. 123.
The method of striking bells
above head.

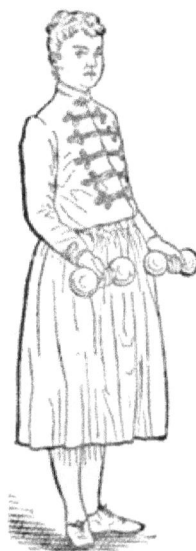

FIG. 124.
Method of striking dumb bells
in front below.

tion the thumb ends may be struck, then the little-finger ends.   From here they swing down and the bells are struck in front below, as seen in Fig. 124, either with thumb or little-finger ends.   When bells are struck back of the body, strike little-finger ends together; but in this case do not bend the body forward (Fig. 125).

The arms may be flexed, the bells held as high as the neck, palms of the hands back, keeping the arms bent ; the little-finger ends, then the thumb ends, can be struck. This makes a good exercise for running or marching.

The " Anvil Strike."—The right bell is placed on the shoulder, thumb down; the left bell is held shoulder-high to the front. (See Fig. 126, pupil on the left, page 123.) With the right bell, strike the left one forcibly, when the left arm swings down, back, and up, and comes to the left shoulder, thumbend down, while the right arm remains front, holding the position that the left one did. This striking motion will require a little practice. The exercise may be reversed. Fig. 126 represents two pupils taking the double " Anvil Strike," in which case the one who strikes, hits her neighbor's bell, and not her own.

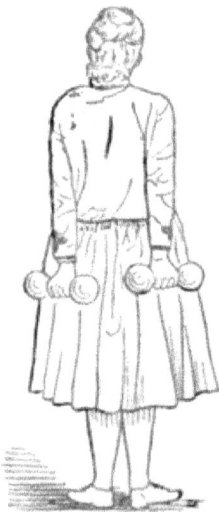

FIG. 125.
Method of striking dumb-bells back below.

Pushing the Dumb-bell.—The bells are on the chest; the right arm is pushed up, palm front; the left bell is brought to the hip; the body inclines to the left, the head thrown slightly back; the face looks up. (See Fig. 127.)

If the teacher thoroughly understands these preliminary movements with the dumb-bells, the following series will be more easily learned and taught. The teacher will perhaps have noticed how the bell is divided into parts : the bulb near the thumb is called the thumb end; that near the little finger, the little-finger end.

First Series.

Position, bells on chest (Fig. 114) ; march time.

I. Thrust the right bell DOWN 4 times, left bell 4, times, both 8 times.

II. Thrust the right bell OUT 4 times, left bell 4 both 8 times.

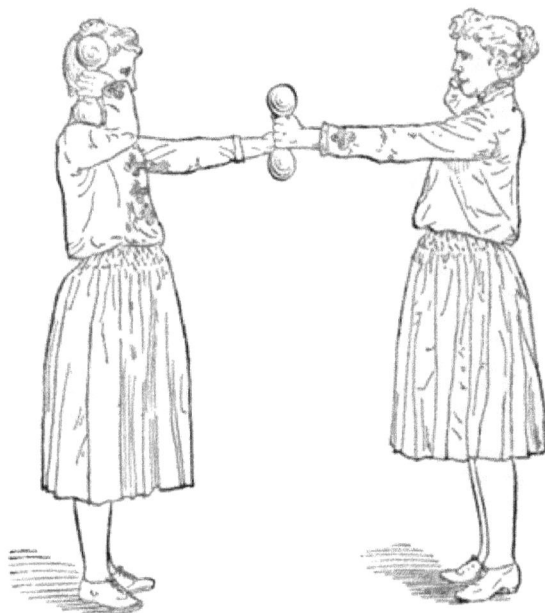

FIG. 126.
Double anvil strike.

III. Thrust the right bell UP 4 times, left up 4, both 8 times.

IV. Thrust the right bell FRONT 4 times, left 4, both 8 times.

V. On the 8th count of the last exercise, bring the bells to the hips.

VI. Bend the body backward and forward, alternating, 8 times.

VII. Bend the body to the right and left sides, alternating, 8 times.

VIII. Swing the right leg to the front and to the right, alternating, 8 times.

IX. Take the same exercise with the left leg. On the 8th count, drop the bells to the side.

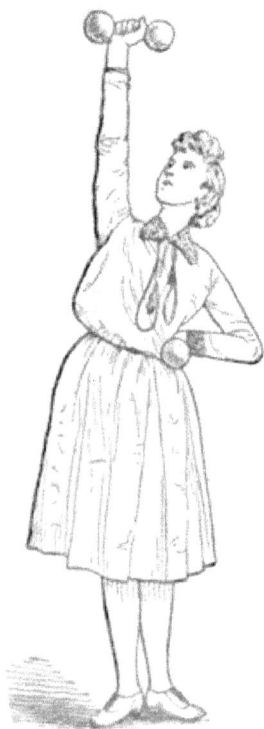

Fig. 127.
Pushing the dumb-bell.

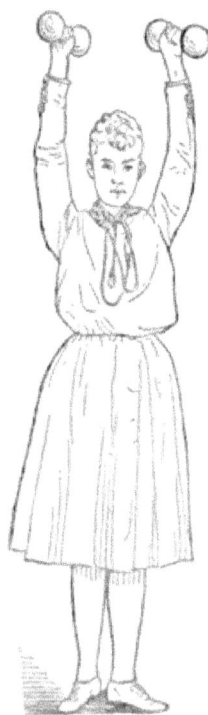

Fig. 128.—Bells up.

X. Flex the right arm 4 times, left 4 times, both 8 times.

XI. Swing the right **arm** shoulder-high **to** the side, 4 times, same with the left, both 8 times.

XII. Swing both bells shoulder-high to the front, palms in, on Count **1**; on **Count** 2, swing **the** hands from this position shoulder-high to the side ; on Counts 3 and 4, strike **the** little-finger ends of the bells together back of **the body.** Take **this** exercise 8 times.

Second Series. Music, March or Waltz Time.

Position, bells on chest.

I. Circle the right bell to the right, **making a heart-shaped circle, as with the** clubs, 8 **times.** (See Fig. **114.)**

II. Circle the **left** bell to the left 8 times. Reverse Nos. I and II, 8 times each.

III. Circle both **bells** to the right 8 times, to the left 8 times.

The circles **I, II, and III** may be alternated, also **reel** and follow **motions** can be made. **See** article on club-swinging.

IV. Thrust **both bells** DOWN, OUT, UP, and FRONT, each 8 times. **On the last 8th count, bring the** bells to the hips.

V. Raise on the toes **16 times; raise the toes 16** times. On last count, drop the bells to the side.

VI. Charge the right foot diagonally forward to **the** right, **and** swing bells above the head 8 times; same with the left. (See Fig. 128 for position of arms.)

Twisting Motions.—These are made by twisting the entire arm so that the palm of **the hand** is first front, **then back.** See description of this exercise. **Of** the 6 twisting motions given, all but one are full-arm motions. (Figs. 120, **121, 122.**)

VII. With the arms **down, twist** the bells 6 times, counting front and back **as one.** On the 7th count bring the bells to the chest, and on 8 thrust the bells OUT. With the bells in this position, proceed as has been described, always **bringing** the bells to the chest on the 7th count. In **a like** manner thrust the arms UP and FRONT, **then** take **a fore-arm twist** (see Fig. 122), and once more **twist** the arms, with **the** bells at **the** side, but do not bring the bells to the chest on 7 (Figs. **120 and 121**).

Third Series. Music, March Time.

Position, bells at the side.

I. **Flex** and straighten the right arm **on** count 1 ; **count 2,** swing the arm, shoulder-high, **to the** side, and lower. Take this exercise 4 times.

II. Take the same with the left hand 4 times ; both 4 times. **On the last 4th** count, bring the bells to the shoulder.

III. Count 1, thrust **the** right hand UP **and bring back to** the shoulder ; count 2, thrust **the** right **hand** OUT **and bring** back **to** the shoulder—8 counts. Same with left arm 8 counts ; both arms 8 counts. On the last 8th count, bring the hands to **the** hips.

IV. Step the right foot *front,* diagonally front to the right, **to** the *right,* and diagonally back **to** the right. Same with the left **foot** and then repeat this exercise. Remember, in **a** stepping motion, to bring the heels together after each step. Sixteen counts.

V. Striking Motions.—Strike the bells in front of the body below; first the thumb ends, then little-finger ends. Sixteen counts (**Fig. 124**).

VI. Strike the bells below, back of the body, same as in front, 16 counts (**Fig 125**).

VII. Strike the bells front and back below, thumb ends in front, little-finger ends back, **16** counts.

In these exercises strike the bells forcibly.

VIII. Right hand *salute* 4 times. This is made by bringing the right bell to the left shoulder, in which case the little-finger end is higher than the thumb end. Left hand "salute" four times. Alternate these motions 8 times (Fig. 116).

IX. Stamp the right foot forcibly 3 times, gaining ground the length of the foot at each stamp, diagonally forward. On the 4th count, bring the heels together. Same with left. Repeat this exercise.

X. Bells on the hips, count 1; on the chest, count 2; on the hips, count 3; at the side on count 4. Take this exercise 4 times. Nos. IX and X can be combined.

XI. On the last exercise of No. X, the bells are brought to the chest, and not to the side; then take the right-angle motions (**Fig. 119**).

XII. Right hand down, left hand out, 4 times; left hand down, right hand out, 4 times; right hand up, left hand out, 4 times; left hand up, right hand out, 4 times.

XIII. "Push the dumb-bell" with the right hand. The right arm is thrust up, palm front, left hand on hip, body inclined to the left, face looking up. (See Fig. 127.) Take 2 counts for pushing the bell up, 2

counts more for bringing the bell to position. Take
the same with the left hand, and repeat the exercise.

XIV. Thrust the right hand front, shoulder-high, on
count 1; on count 2, without moving the feet, thrust
the right arm back, shoulder-high, and look in the

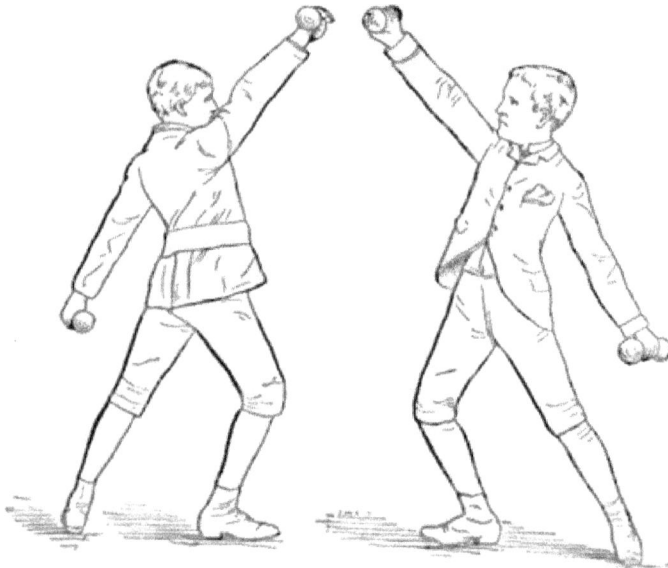

Fig. 129.
" A simple attitude."

same direction, 8 counts. Same with the left hand
8 counts.

On the 8th count, bring the bells under the arms,
swing right hand out, shoulder-high, to the side, palm
down, 4 times; same with left 4 times; both bells 8
times (Fig 130). On 8th count, bring the bells to the
shoulders (Fig. 131).

XV. Charge to the right, and thrust right hand out,

shoulder-high, to the side 4 times. Same on left 4 times. On the 8th count, drop the hands to the sides.

A few statues can be given to finish this exercise,— Boxer, Gladiator, Putting the Shot, etc.,—or the series may be finished by the Anvil Chorus.

MARCHING SERIES.

It affords a pleasant variety if the dumb-bell exercises can be taken while the pupils are marching

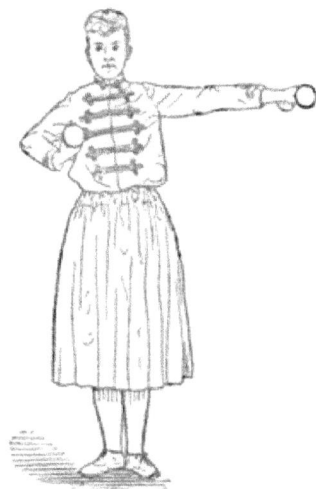 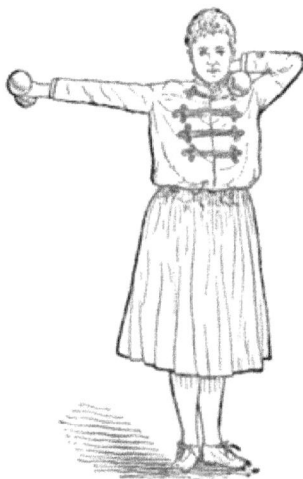

FIG. 130.   FIG. 131.

FIG. 130.—Method of thrusting bell from **under** the shoulder out. **The** right hand shows the bell under the shoulder, the left **hand the bell when thrust** out.

FIG. 131.—The left hand rests on the shoulder, **the right hand** shows position when the bell is thrust out.

around the room. The following series can be given, and they will be found not only pleasing, but valuable.

If the sexes exercise together, it is well to have the boys march in one direction and the girls in another.

Striking Series.

I. Strike **the** thumb ends **of** the bells in front on the first of each 4 counts for 16 or **32** steps.

II. Strike the little-finger ends **of the** bells back on the first of each **4** counts.

III. Strike **the** bells in front **on 1, back on 3.**

IV. Strike the **bells** front and back below **on every** count, **thumb** ends in **front,** little-finger ends **back.**

V. Flex **the** arms, **back of** the hands to the **front,** bells height **of the neck; strike the** bells together **on** each count, first the little-finger, then the **thumb, ends.** This exercise can be **taken** with the run, **whether in place** or around the room. **Let the class take the** marching series while they **mark time.**

Second Marching Series.

To slow march time or ordinary waltz time, take the circling **and** thrusting motions of **the** Second Series of the dumb-bells. **There is** a change to quicker time after the circling motions in this series.

Third Marching Series.

Take, to **ordinary march** time, the exercises I, II, III, V, VI, VII, **VIII, X, XI,** XII of **the Third** Series of Dumb-bells.

If the gymnasium is small, omit, **in the** Marching Series, all motions where the hands **are** thrust OUT or FRONT.

Many exercises **for** wands and free gymnastics can be taken to march time.

ANVIL CHORUS.

This is an exercise, arranged with dumb-bells, set to the Anvil Chorus from "Il Trovatore." The time of the music is common, there being four beats to the measure. In the description of the exercise, a count and one beat is the same.

I. Counts 1 and 2, bells on the hips (Fig. 113); 3 and 4, bells at the side (Fig. 112); 1 and 2, bells on chest (Fig. 114); 3 and 4, at the side; 1 and 2, bells at the back (Fig. 117); 3 and 4, at the side; 1 and 2, bells on shoulders (Fig. 115); 3 and 4, at side. Repeat this exercise.

II. Counts 1 and 2, charge right foot diagonally forward; 3 and 4, bring heels together and right face; 1 and 2, charge right foot diagonally back; 3 and 4, heels together and front face. Take same exercise on the left side. Repeat this exercise. Keep the hands on the hips.

III. Counts 1 and 2, bring the right foot back of the left, toes on the floor, heels up (see Fig. 34); on 3 and 4, execute an about face and bring the heels together. Next four counts, execute another about face to the right, coming back to the first position, and drop the bells to the side.

IV. Counts 1 and 2, charge the right foot diagonally forward, curve right arm over head, left arm back of the body (see Fig. 132); 3 and 4, come back to position. Same attitude on the left side. Repeat this exercise.

V. On 1 and 2, right face and bring bells to the

hips; 3 and 4, front face, bells at the side.   Same on left.   On the last count, bring the right bell to the right shoulder, hold the left bell shoulder-high to the front.   This position is seen in Fig. 126, pupil on the left.

VI. Anvil Strike.—Strike the left bell with the right, swing the left bell down, back, and around to the left shoulder, while the right bell remains shoulder-high to the front.   The position is now the same as in the figure, except that the right hand is front and the left hand is on the shoulder. 'Continue this striking exercise through 8 counts; drop bells at side on the 8th count.

VII. Strike the bells above the head (Fig. 123) and shoulder-high in front, alternating; take this for 8 counts.   Do not strike the bells when they are down.

VIII. Strike the bells front and back below, 8 counts, which makes 16 clicks with the bells.

IX. Charge the right foot diagonally forward and strike the bells above the head; come to position and strike the bells back below (Fig. 125); then strike front and back below; same on the left side.   Repeat this exercise.   This will make 16 clicks.

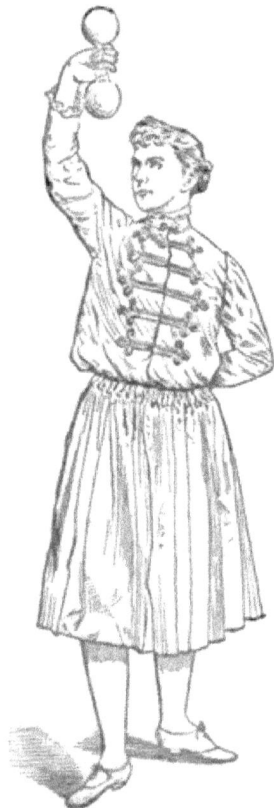

FIG. 132.
A simple attitude.

X. Interlude.—Counts 1 and 2, bells on the chest (Fig. 114); 3 and 4, bells OUT (Fig. 133), palms front; 5 and 6, bells UP (Fig. 128), but do not strike; 7 and 8, bells FRONT (Fig. 134); 9 and 10, shoulder-high to

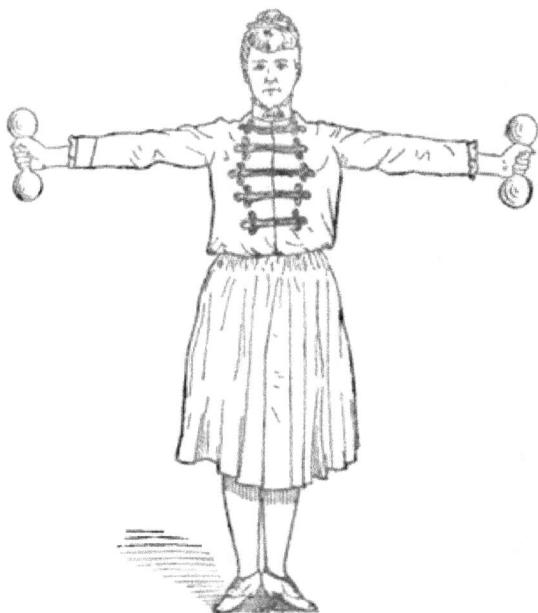

FIG. 133.
Bells out, or shoulder-high to the side.

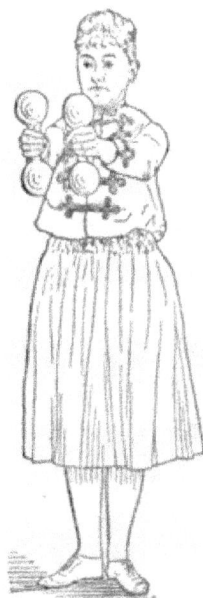

FIG. 134.
Bells front.

the side or OUT (Fig. 133); 11 and 12, bells down (Fig. 112); on count 13, strike the bells sharply in front below. In this exercise the bells pass from one position to another, but do not come to the chest.

XI. Stamping Motions.—On 1 and 2, stamp right foot twice, gaining ground the length of the foot on each step; on 3, heels together, and strike the bells smartly back of the body. Take the same exercise on the left side.

XII. Finish.—Counts 1 and 2, strike bells in front below; **3 and 4,** charge right foot diagonally forward and strike bells above the head; 5 and 6, bring the **feet to** the position of an officer's about face, the same as in exercise **No.** 34; same time, strike bells back below; 7 and 8, **kneel** right knee **to** the floor and strike bells over the **head. Come to** the position at a **chord.**

A special **arrangement of the** music for the Anvil Chorus will **be sent by the** author to any address.

PIZZICATI CHORUS (SINGLE FORM).

An arrangement **with the** dumb-bells **set to the** Pizzicati, from the opera **"Sylvia."** Position, **bells at side.**

I. Count 1, right bell **on chest; 2, left bell on the chest;** 3, thrust the right **bell OUT; 4, the left bell; 5,** strike bells above the head; **6, strike bells back** below; **7, front below; 8,** rest the bells **at** the side. This exercise taken rapidly 3 times. (First striking motion.)

II. Count 1, stamp right foot diagonally forward; **2,** click the bells **in front** of that leg; 3, bring **the heels** together; 4, strike the bells back. Take **the same** exercise **on** the left side. (First stamping **motion.)**

III. Count 1, bells OUT, palms of the hands **up; 2,** bring bells to shoulder; 3, bells OUT; 4, strike bells UP; **5,** bells OUT; 6, strike bells FRONT; 7, strike bells back below; 8, rest the bells at **the** side. Take this exercise three times. (Second striking motion.)

IV. Count 1, stamp right foot diagonally front; 2, heels together; 3, stamp left foot diagonally forward; and 4, heels together; on 5, 6, **and 7,** strike the "rataplan," and rest the bells at the side on 8. (Second stamping motion.)

The "Rataplan" is made by bending the arms until the fore-arms are parallel to the floor (Fig. 122), the palms of the hands towards each other. Now, by twisting both fore-arms to the left, the thumb end of the right bell will strike the little-finger end of the left bell. This takes one count. By twisting the fore-arms to the right, the strike is made with the left thumb and right little-finger ends of the bells. This striking exercise, kept up for several counts, is called the "rataplan." Unless otherwise stated, there will be but three clicks of the bells, and the hands will rest at the side on the 4th or 8th count.

V. On beats 1 and 2, take the posture seen in Fig. 132; on 3 and 4, come back to position. Take this exercise 3 times, and make the rataplan as described.

VI. Take posture (see Fig. 135); on 1 and 2, charge left foot diagonally back; extend and elevate right hand, palm down, left bell on the hip; 3 and 4, come back to position. Take this position 3 times and one rataplan; notice, in these postures, the position of the head; the face is generally raised.

VII. Counts 1 and 2, charge right foot to the right, right arm out, left arm up (right angle), look to the right; 3 and 4, come to position. Take this exercise 3 times, and make one rataplan. Notice in Fig. 136 the position of the hands.

VIII. The same as exercise No. VII, but taken on the left side.

IX. On 1 and 2, strike the bells once above the

head ; 3 and 4, strike the bells once back below ; 5 and
6, strike once front below ; 7 and 8, strike once back
below again ; 9 and 10, strike the bells front ; counts

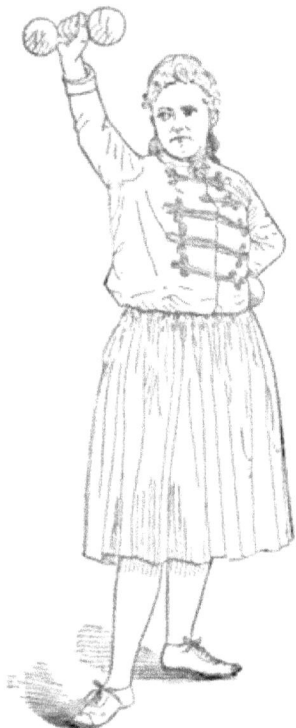

Fig. 135.
A simple attitude.

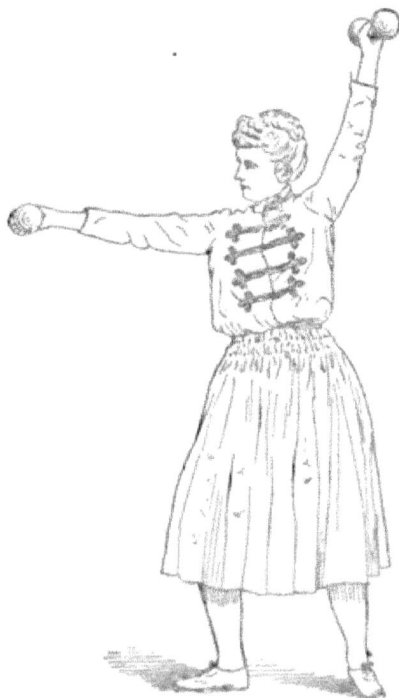

Fig. 136.
Right-angle motion combined with
the charge to the right.

11, 12, 13, 14, 15, 16 are the same as ·3, 4, 5, 6, 7, 8.
Repeat this exercise. These 32 counts are taken to
quick time.

X. The same as No. III, to slower time than
for IX.

XI. The same as No. IV.

The music for this arrangement of the dumb-bells can be had from the author.

PIZZICATI CHORUS (DOUBLE FORM).

This exercise will be found more difficult than the single form. It is necessary there should be an even number of scholars in the class, who are standing upon footmarks 6 or 7 feet apart. We will deal with two lines only. Proceed as in the Single Form of the Pizzicati, up to exercise **IV**, when at count 1 the one on the right charges forward with the left foot, the one on the left charges forward with the right foot. (We shall speak of these feet hereafter as the "inside feet;" of those that remain in place as the "outside feet." In a like manner we will distinguish the arms.)

Count 2, strike the bells in front; count 3, bring the outside foot up to the inside foot; count 4, strike the bells back of the body; make the rataplan. It will now be seen that the two lines are brought closer together; if not close enough, the first charge can be made more to the left and right.

V. Take the posture seen in Fig. 132, charging forward with the inside foot, and curve the inside arm over the head 3 times; rataplan, or take Fig. 129.

VI. Take the second posture (Fig. 135), the two lines charging away from each other with the outside foot, but extending and elevating the inside arm. On the last count, bring the bells to the chest.

VII. Make the *right-angle motions*, the lines charging towards each other 3 times; one rataplan. In this exercise, those on the right thrust the arm back of those on the left, but turn palm of inside hand front (Fig. 136).

VIII. Take the *right-angle motions*, the lines charging away from each other ; rataplan. **On the** 4th count, the lines face each other and take the position seen in Fig. 126. This striking motion **has been** described in the **Anvil** Chorus ; but in this case the pupil does not strike **his own** bell, **but** that of his neighbor. Take this striking exercise 8 times to rapid music, 4 counts to each **stroke. On** the **32d** count, the pupils face front, quickly step away from each other by a side **step,** and finish the series as has been described **in the Single Form.**

CHAPTER X.

CLUB-SWINGING.

Circles, short and long.

Directions, right and left, front and back.

Time, double, follow, reel.

Location.

Short Circles: 1, shoulder; 2, lower front; 3, lower back ; 4, overhead. With the arm extended, the short circles can be made head-, shoulder-, elbow-, and hip-high to the side.

A Long **Circle** is modified to a heart-shaped circle.

Complete Circles are combinations of short and heart-shaped circles.

Combinations are the result of combining the different varieties of complete circles. They are very numerous, and may be made easy or hard. . In this chapter we shall deal only with the simple combinations.

A Pass.—When pupils are beginning their exercises in club-swinging, it is customary to use but one club ; and that there may be **as few** stops as possible while exercising, children should be drilled in passing **their** clubs from one hand to the other.

EXPLANATORY.

In plain club-swinging, we make use of but two kinds of circles—a long or full-arm, and a short or

139

wrist, circle. All evolutions made by the clubs are
parts or variations of these two.

The principal modification of a long circle is seen
in Fig. 137, where the club, instead of continuing in

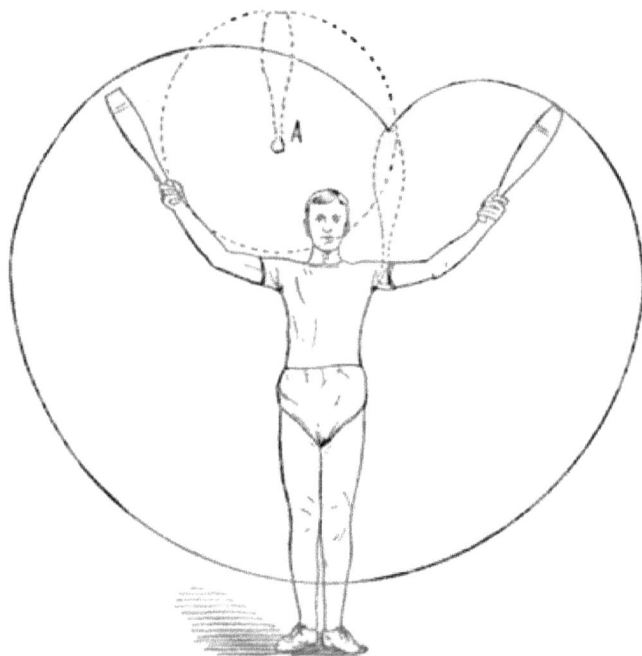

FIG. 137.

FIG. 137 illustrates the single and double heart-shaped circles **out.** **The club**
at the point *A* outlines the short circle **overhead.** Notice that **the club** passes in
front of the face.

a perfect circle, is brought back **to the** position of rest.
By looking at **the** outline of this **turn,** it resembles
somewhat a heart, and is therefore appropriately called
the "heart-shaped" circle.

Until this simple evolution is properly learned, **a**
pupil cannot swing clubs well. The club, in going to

the right, should not swing to the front or back of the
shoulder, but should describe a circle passing through
the center and to the right of the shoulder. Or, the
club should swing along the central line on the body

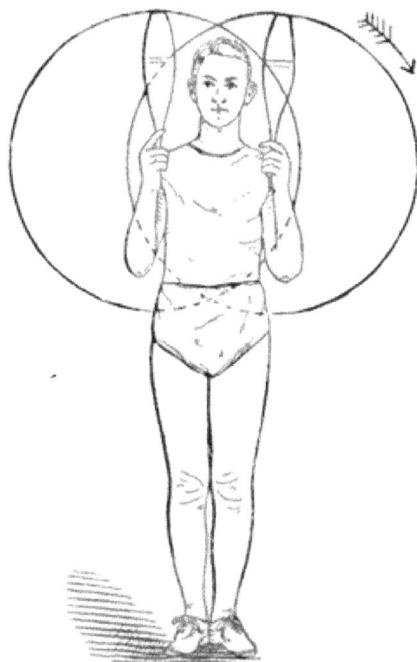

Fig. 138.

Fig. 138 shows the first position in club-swinging. The outlines indicate the
short shoulder-circles out.

of the pupil standing to the right of the club-swinger.
This is an important rule.

Again, the circle must be made with the full arm,
and not with the fore-arm. It will be seen that pupils
with close-fitting waist garments resort to the fore-arm
circles too frequently; and while executing such a

circle, the elbow is only moved a trifle.   Urge the
pupils to move their elbows.

Long Circles and heart-shaped circles are made

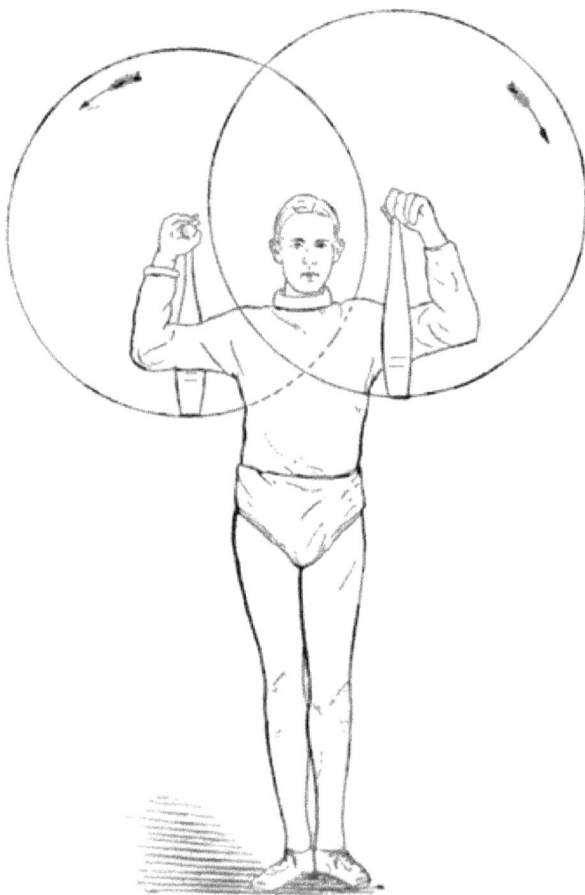

Fig. 133.

The right hand illustrates **a short** shoulder circle to the right back of the
shoulder. The circle made by **the left** hand is the front shoulder-circle, or
circle in front of the shoulder to the left.   It will be easy to change from one circle to the other; moreover, it can be quickly learned if the full arm circles in the
reel, seen in Fig. 143, are changed to wrist motions as shown in this illustration.

to the right and left; to the FRONT, and to the REAR.

A Short Circle (Fig. 138) is much more difficult to teach and to learn.

The club is held loosely in the hand, grasped by the thumb and first two fingers. In executing the turn, give the arm as much play as it requires. Remember, that in handling clubs, the arms are not to be restricted too much.

The short circle back of the shoulder is made to the right, or OUT, and reversed (see Fig. 138). The short circle *in front* of the shoulder is made to the right and reversed (Fig. 139, left hand). The short circles at the shoulder are made to the front and reversed, or to the rear (Fig. 140).

These circles are made

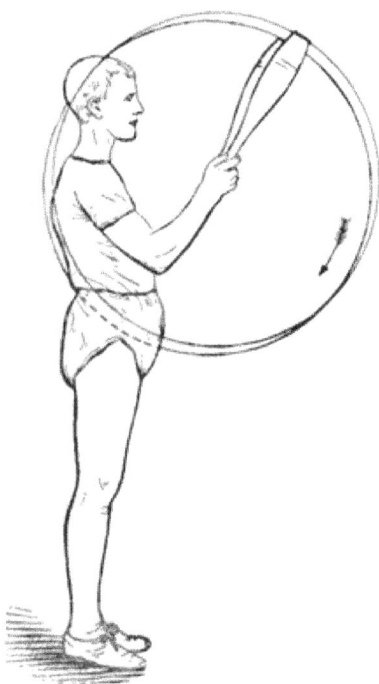

Fig. 140.
A double shoulder-circle to **the front.**

with both clubs going in the same direction (Fig. 141), or in different directions (Fig. 138).

To teach a short shoulder-circle in any direction, it is well to direct the class to drop the club one quarter of a circle in that direction 16 or 24 times, until they have a definite idea of which way it is to go. The

short shoulder-circle to the front is the easiest of this
class, and should be taught first (Fig. **140**).   The front
shoulder-circles to the right or left should **be** taught
last.   They are not easily mastered.   Short circles are

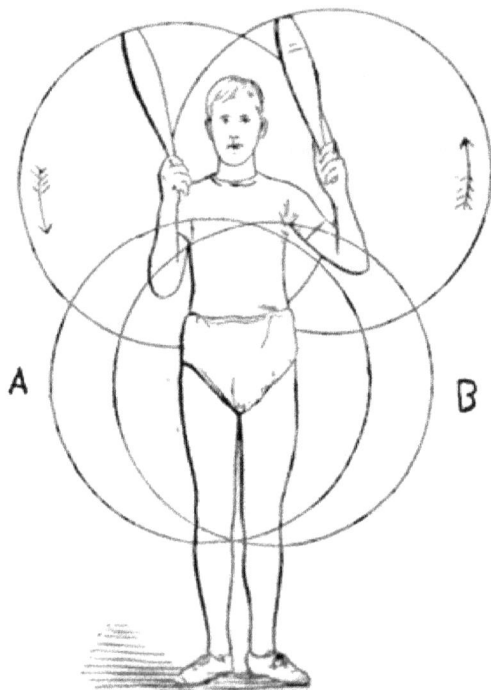

Fig. 141.

Fig 141 shows a double shoulder-circle to the right   The circles *A* and *B* outline the lower front   In this position the arm **is** slightly bent, the hand being a
little lower than the hip.

made at arm's length overhead (Fig. 137 *A*), or they
may **be** made shoulder-high **to** the side, DOWN in front
of the body or "lower front" (Fig. 141 *A* and *B*),
DOWN back of **the** body or "lower back" (Fig.

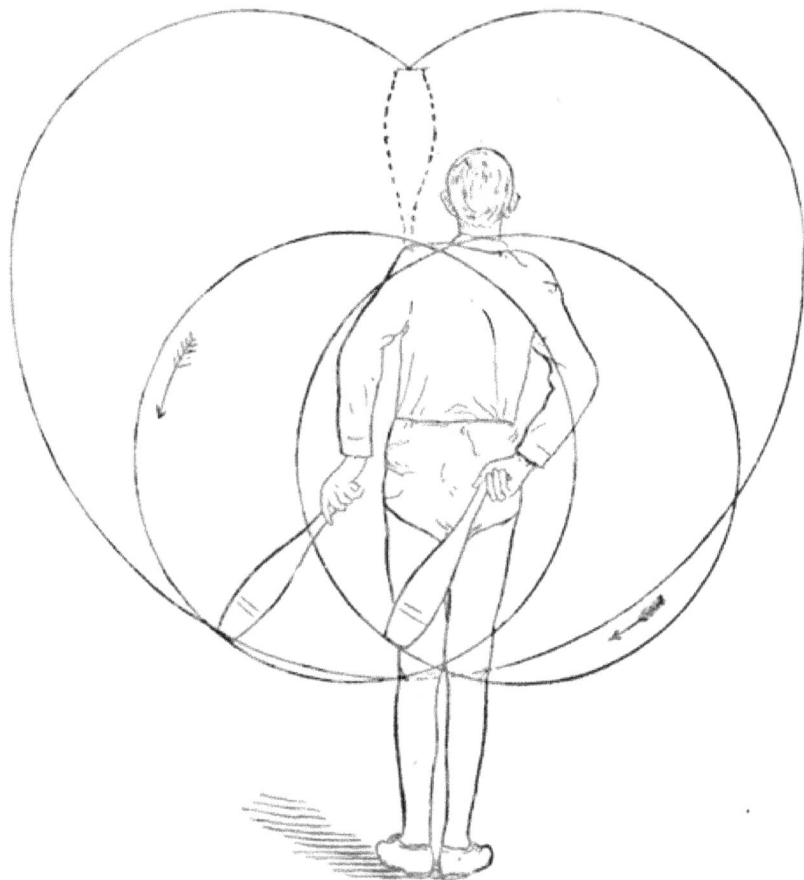

FIG. 142.

By following the course of the club in the left hand, we trace the outline of a complete back-circle. Notice that the palm of the hand will point in the direction that the club is going. The right-hand club goes in an opposite direction.

142). The last is the most difficult of these circles.

Circles are single when made with one club, or double when made with two. They are made to three kinds of time.

Time.

1. "Parallels" when the two clubs go in similar directions and keep the same time, beginning and finishing together (Fig. 141).

2. "Follows" where one club starts and the second

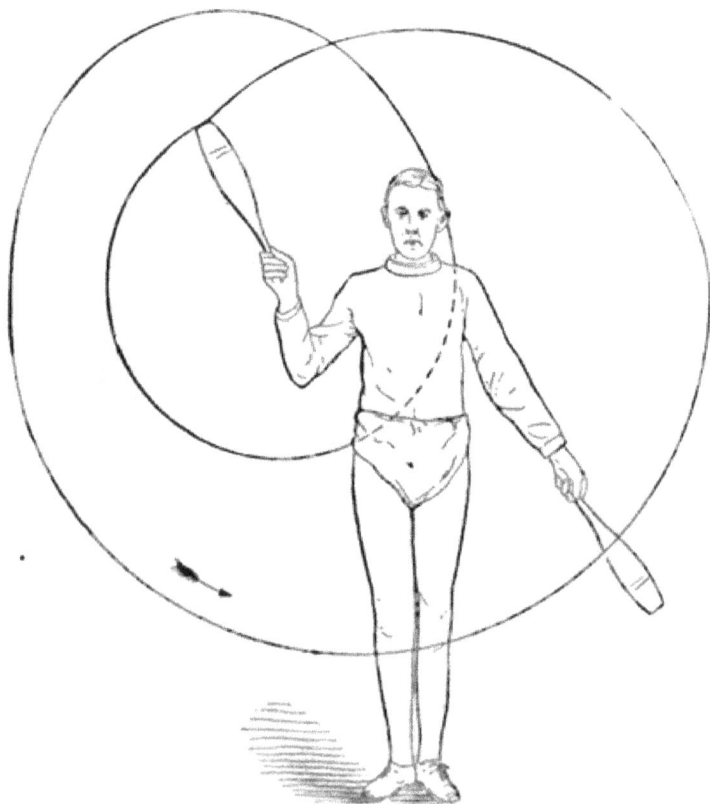

Fig. 143.

Fig. 143 illustrates the "reel." The outline of the right club is given; that of the left is the same, although not shown in the cut. Both clubs are executing the same maneuver, but the one club is half a circle ahead of the other. In this circle the rhythm is most even. The outline indicated by the right hand is that of a complete shoulder-circle to the right.

club follows, whether in the same or in different directions. The clubs neither start nor finish at the same time, but one follows the other. They are about one third of a circle apart (Fig. 144).

3. "Reels" are similar to Follows, but the cadence is more even. The clubs are one half of a circle apart. "Reel," as a name, however, is only given to the combination of the complete shoulder circles *out* and reversed (Fig. 143).

With this may be combined the "overhead," the "lower front," and "back" circles.

"The Reels" are the smoothest of all turns (Fig. 143); one club makes a short, while the other makes the heart-shaped part of the complete circle.

Position.—In every respect that of a soldier, but the arms must be flexed, the hands grasp the clubs not too tightly, the clubs perpendicular and about the width of the shoulders apart. (See Fig. 138.)

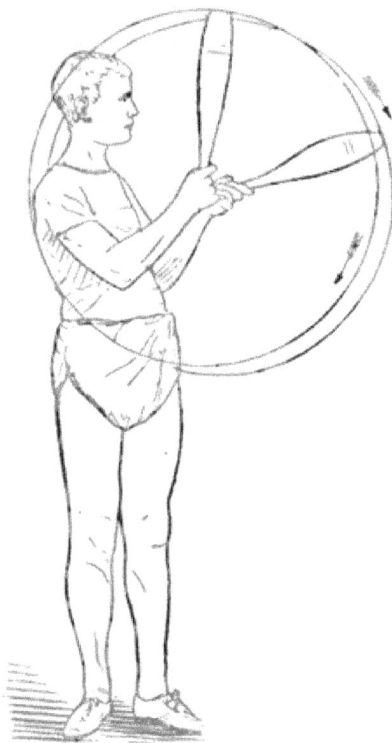

FIG. 144.

FIG. 144 illustrates "follow" time. It will be seen that one club starts ahead of the other. Both clubs do not finish the exercise at the same time, but one follows the other.

A Long Circle.—Raise the club, kept in a vertical position, to full arm's length above the head. Now, without bending the arm but a very little, execute a long circle to the right or left, with the shoulder as a pivot. This can be taken any number of times, the club being brought to position on the last count.

A Double **Long** Circle is executed with both clubs to the right or to the left.

A Double **Outside Circle** is executed by swinging the right club to the right, and the left club to the left,

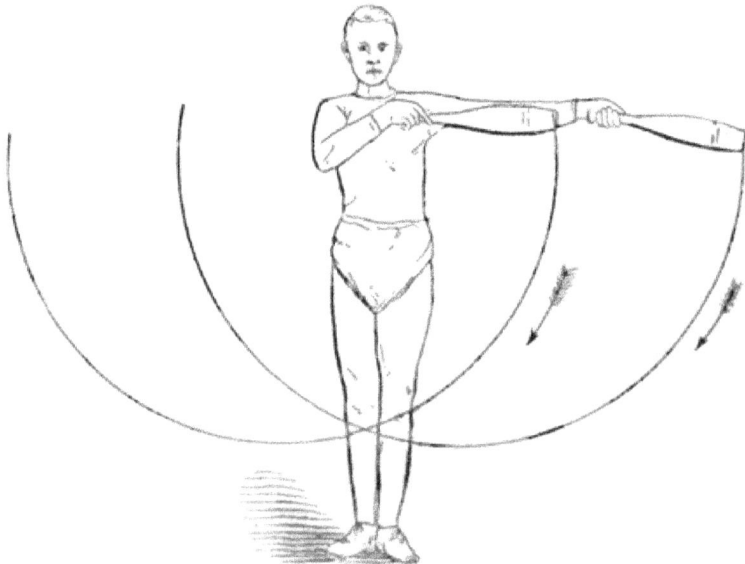

FIG. 145.
A side pendulum from right to left.

simultaneously. This may be reversed. Long circles may also be executed to reel or follow time. They may be made to the front and rear.

A Pendulum is half a long circle. The clubs swing

from right to left and from left to right, going only
shoulder-high on each side. Keep the shoulders to the
front (Fig. 145). The pendulum can be made from front
to rear (Fig. 146).

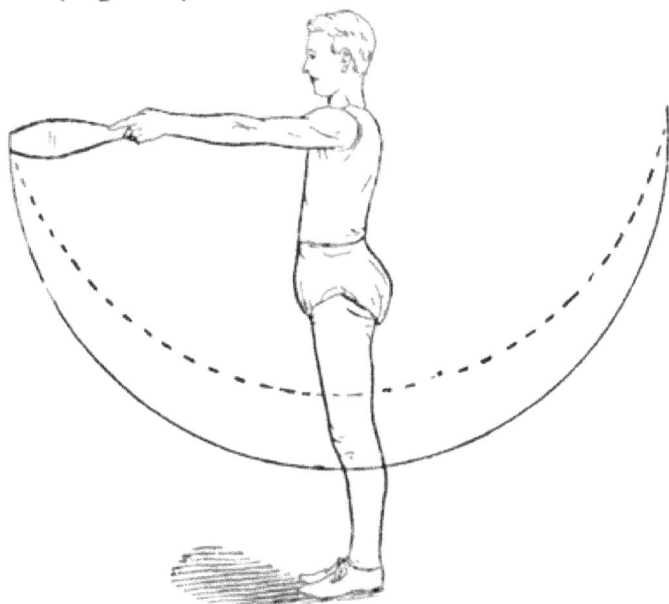

FIG. 146.
A pendulum from front to rear.

Short Circles—At the Shoulder.—A double back-circle
to the right or left is when both clubs swing back of
the shoulder to the right or left (Fig. 141). A double
circle to the front is when both clubs swing to the
front (Fig. 140). These may be reversed.

A "Drop" circle to the right is when the shoulders
are turned to the right without moving the feet, and
both clubs swing in that direction. This circle can
be made shoulder-high, elbow-high, and hip-high on
each side.

A Double Outside Circle is when the right club goes to the right and the left to the left. This may be **reversed.**

A Double Short Circle in front of the shoulders, to the right or left, is made by flexing the arms, palms of the hands front, and by making with the hand and knob of the club a "ball-and-socket" joint, then swinging the clubs to **the right or** left in *front* of the shoulders **(Fig. 139, left hand).** This is a difficult exercise. Teachers will **notice** the difference between a *front* shoulder-circle and a circle to the **front.**

The short circles **at** the shoulder **can be made to double,** follow, or reel time.

Lower Front.—The **club** swings from position **down below** the waist; the arm is stopped at the **side, but** the **club** continues its motion, and by using **the wrist** as **a pivot a** circle is made as seen **in** Fig. **141** *A* and *B.* Do **not** grasp the **club** too firmly. After the short circle has been **made,** continue with a heart-shaped circle, and come **back to** position or make a pendulum to the left. Swing back to the right and reverse **the** lower front. The double lower front can **be** made **to** the right or left. These circles can **be made to reel** or follow time.

Lower Back.—These are considered **the** most difficult **of** all circles. They should **not be** taught until **the** other circles are learned. **As** in the lower front, swing **the** club from position *down,* stop the arm partly bent, at the side, but permit the club to make a short circle back of **the** body; when finished, bring the club **to the** front and continue with **a** full circle, or make a pendulum and reverse the lower back. In this circle the palm of the hand should face the way the club turns. The arm should be bent to such a degree that the end of the club is seen above the shoulder. The club does not pass *between* the arm and back in this circle. The circles can be single or double, outside and reversed, to follow and reel time.

Overhead.—Make a long circle, but when the arm is up stop it, and let the club continue until it completes the short circle over the head. The knob of the club and the thumb and first two fingers make a " ball-and-socket " joint. Much practice is required to make good overhead circles. They are made in the same direction and to the same time as other short circles. (See Fig. 137 *A.*)

Complete Circles are made by combining long and short or " heart-shaped " and short circles. The description of the following complete circles will apply to any complete circles.

A complete back shoulder-circle to the right is made by a heart-shaped circle to the right, and without a stop, executing a short shoulder-circle to the right in combination. This may be reversed. (Fig. 143.)

These circles may be single or double, outside or reverse. The complete circle at the shoulder can be made to the front or rear (Fig. 147). Complete circles in front of the shoulders are made and executed on the same principle as the complete back shoulder-circles.

The following complete circles will be understood by referring to the figures :

A complete lower-front (Fig. 141 *A*).

A complete lower-back (Fig. 142).

A complete overhead (Fig. 137 *A*).

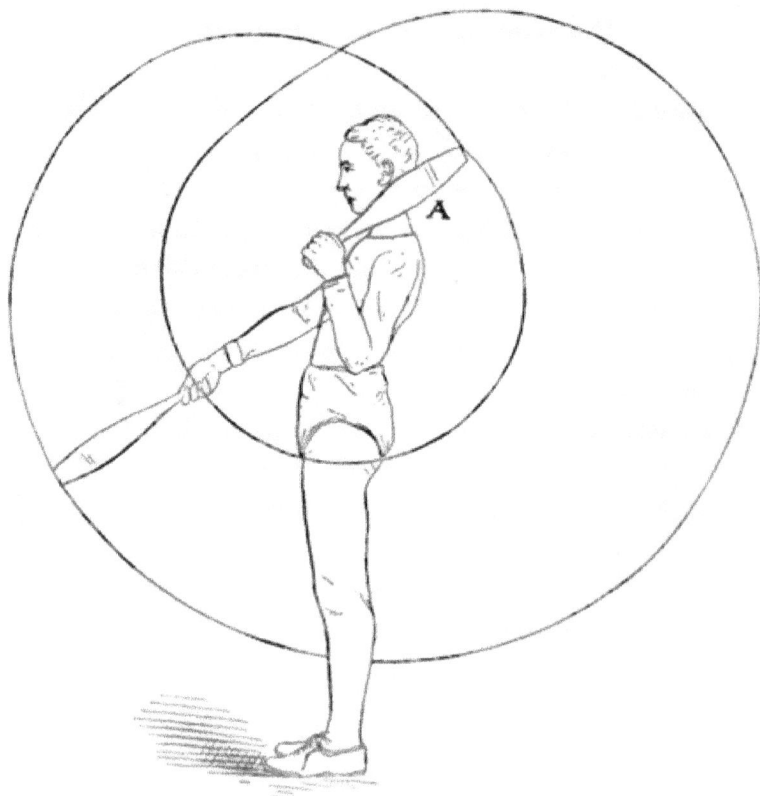

Fig. 147.

Fig. 147 illustrates a reel combination of the shoulder-circles to the front   The outline followed by the club *A* is that of a complete shoulder-circle to the front.

A few exercises with the clubs that cannot be classified under the circles already described :

1st. Overhead parallels.

2d. Drops.

3d. Raises.

4th. Horizontal circles.

The Overhead Parallel is made by swinging the club from position out to the right, down in front and up

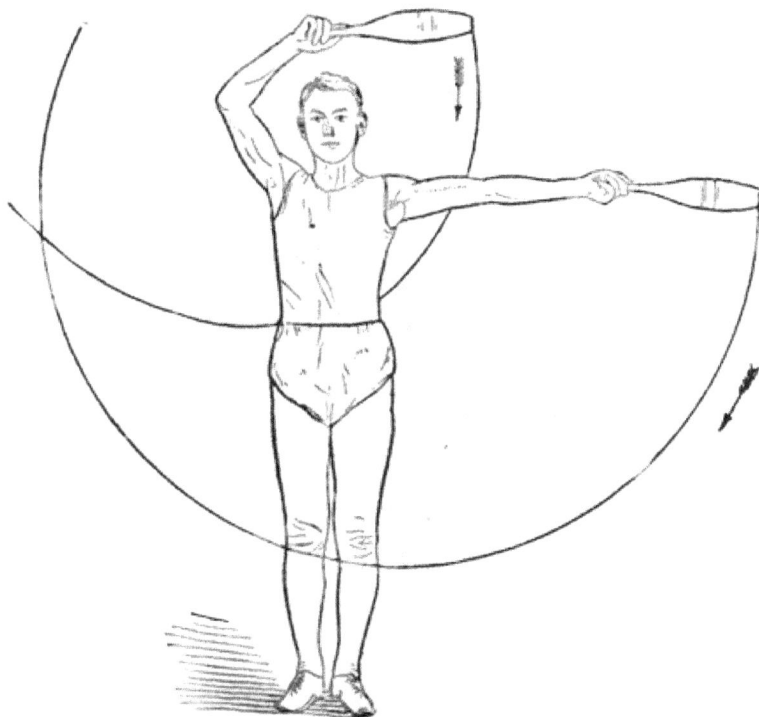

FIG. 148.

FIG. 148 represents the double overhead parallel. Notice that the club overhead drops back of the body while the extended club makes a pendulum to the opposite side.

over the head until it is parallel to the floor. (See Fig. 148.) It is then dropped down back of the head,

passes the shoulders, and extended full arm's length
to the right, where it is again parallel to the floor.
(See left hand, Fig. 148.) From this **position repeat**

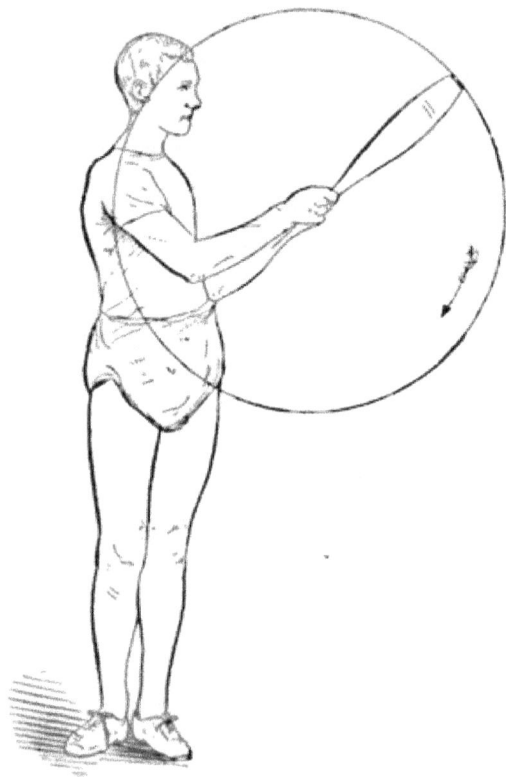

FIG. 149.

Fig. 149 is the start for drop-circle; both shoulders turn to the left, both clubs
point the same way. After the short circles make a pendulum and swing to the
right, and take the same on that side.

the exercise. When taken **with** both clubs, the club
above the head and that at arm's length are both par-
allel to the floor at the same time. The overhead
club is dropped back of the head as the extended club
makes the pendulum part of the swing.

Reverse.—The extended arm, instead of swinging in front of the body, is brought back of the shoulder by flexing the arm, and passed up and over the head and then dropped down in front and out to extended position.

The Drop is a combination of the pendulum and a double shoulder-circle to the right and left. Start from position, turn the shoulders to right or left, make a double shoulder-circle to the right or left (Fig. 149), then a pendulum to the right or left; stop the clubs when extended arm's length to the left, and when parallel to the floor. From this position make a double short circle to the left (Fig. 149), then a pendulum, and back to the right.

In this exercise do not move the feet.

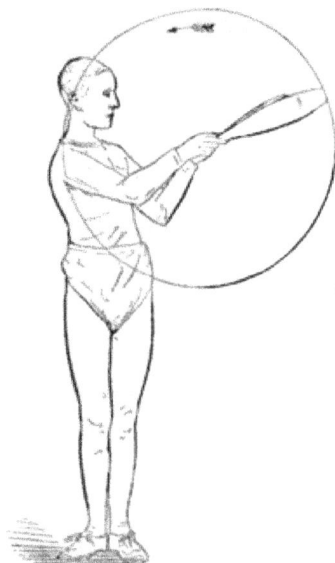

Fig. 150.

Fig. 150 is the reverse of Fig. 148. It will be seen that the clubs, instead of dropping to are raised from the floor, going in the direction of the arrow. After finishing the circle, make a pendulum and execute the same on the right side.

A Raise.—It will be noticed that in the drop, when the clubs are parallel to the floor, the ends drop or swing down (Fig. 149). Now instead of dropping the ends of the clubs, raise them and reverse the *drop* by making a short circle in the opposite direction (Fig. 150). When the circle is finished the clubs are in starting position (parallel to the floor). Now make the pendulum to the right (or left), and take the same on that side.

The Inside Raise and Inside Drop are made by letting the clubs swing inside of the arms and not outside.

A Horizontal Circle (on the right).— Swing the clubs up to the *drop* position on the right. Instead of executing a raise or drop, the points of the clubs pass away from each other and execute short wrist-circles parallel to the floor. (See Fig. 151.) Next make a pendulum and take the same on the left. The short part of this circle can be reversed. A very pretty combination of this circle is seen in Fig. 152. Shoulders front. The right arm extended across in front of the body to the left, club parallel to the floor. Now swing the arm from left to right, keeping the hand shoulder-high; at the same time make a single horizontal circle. **This** circle can be made with both hands going from right to left or left to right, but in both cases in the horizontal circles, the ends of the clubs swing front. The circle can be made to reel time.

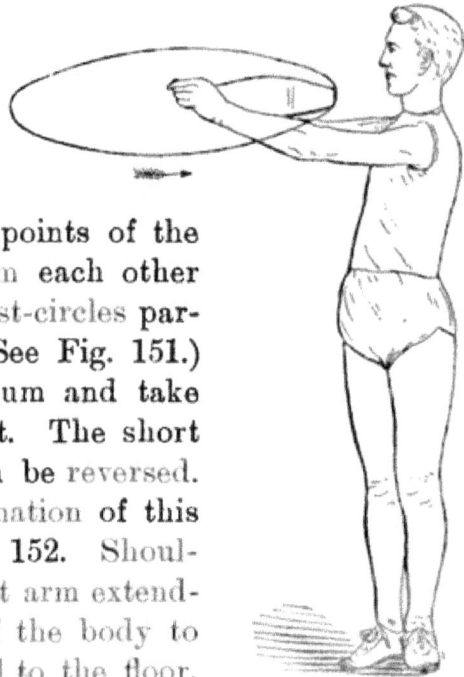

FIG 151.

Fig. 151 represents side or horizontal circles. In the starting position the clubs point out, and are parallel to the floor. The points of the clubs pass away from each other, back and roll over the fore arms as shown by the arrow. After this execute a pendulum, and take the same on the other side.

The author gives this series to children between the ages of 6 and 8 years, after they have been drilled in the Second Series with the bells. Position, see Fig. 138. Music, waltz time.

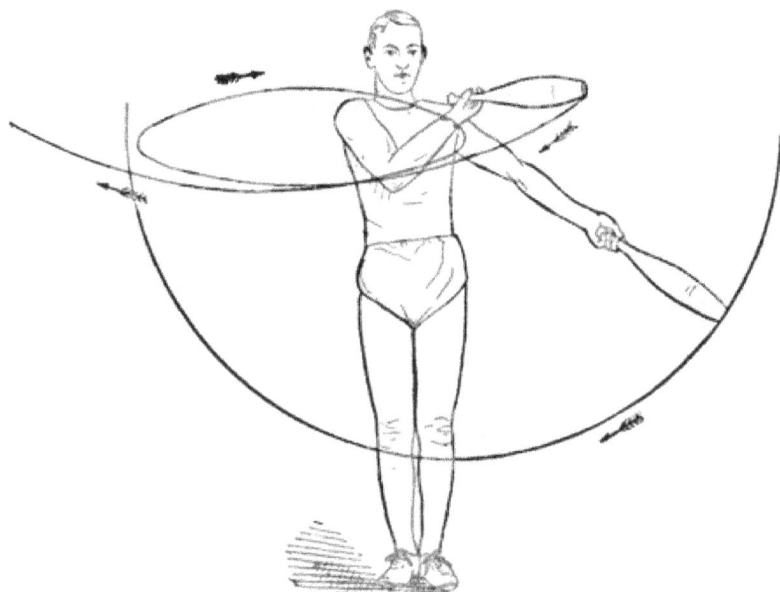

Fig. 152.

Fig. 152 shows a combination of the horizontal circles; the right hand follows the outline indicated by the arrows, while the left hand is supposed to have finished the same circle, and is making a pendulum motion to the right side to a position similar to that held by the right hand. The right hand, after executing the side circle, makes a pendulum.

1. Heart-shaped circle with right hand to the right 4 times.

2. Reverse 4 times; pass.

3. Same exercises with the left hand, and pass.

4. Pendulum from left to right 16 **times.** On the 16th **count,** stop the club **at** the side.

5. Pendulum from front to rear 16 times, **and pass.**

6. Take the pendulum exercises with the left hand in the same manner, and pass the club back ; bring **to** position.

7. Make a **quarter** of a **short** shoulder-circle to the front **8** times **and to the** right **8** times ; pass **to left** hand and take the same exercise ; **pass.**

8. Make short shoulder-circles **to the front, and pass** ; **take the** same with the left hand.

9. Drill the pupils on the first complete shoulder-circle **in** club-swinging.

CLUBS.

First Series.   Waltz, or March Time.

For position, **see** Fig. 138.

1. Right club, heart-shaped **circle** to the right 8 times (Fig. **137,** left hand).

2. Left **club to the** left 8 times.

3. Right club to the left 8 times.

4. Left club **to** the right 8 times.

5. Double heart-shaped circle to the right **8** times, and reverse 8 times.

6. Short shoulder-circle **to** the right with the right club (Fig. 138).

7. Short shoulder-circle with the left club to the left **8** times (Fig. 138).

8. Reverse right club 8 times ; reverse left **club** 8 times.

9. Right club, complete shoulder-circle to the right 8 times (Fig. 143).

10. Left club, complete shoulder-circle to the left 8 times.

11. Reverse Nos. 9 and 10, 8 times each.

12. Right club lower front and reverse, combine with the pendulum ; on the 8th count, stop the club at the side.

13. Left hand lower front and reverse 8 times ; on 8th count, make a double pendulum from left to right ; on the next 8th count, make an overhead parallel (Fig. 148) with the right club ; on 8th count again, bring the right club to the side and raise the left club shoulder-high to the left ; with the left club, make the overhead parallel 7 times ; on the 8th count, bring both clubs to position. Make the drop circle combined with the pendulum 8 times ; on the 8th count, make a half-pendulum and bring the clubs to position (Fig. 138).

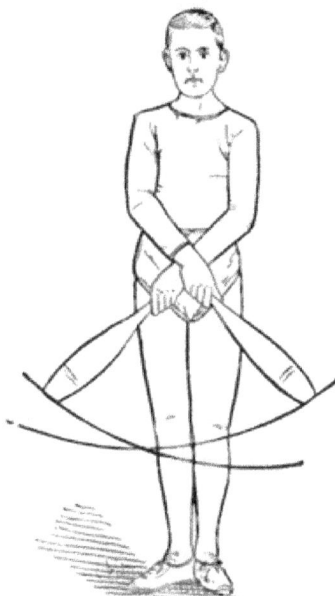

FIG. 153.

Fig. 153 illustrates the method of passing the hands in a double outside heart-shaped circle.

Make 8 double short shoulder-circles to the front (Fig. 140), and catch the clubs under the arms on the 4th count (see Fig. 154).

In this series, the heart-shaped circles and the shoulder circles can be alternated.

Series 1, 2, and 3 are arranged for music. This will account for certain irregularities in the number of times the exercises are taken.

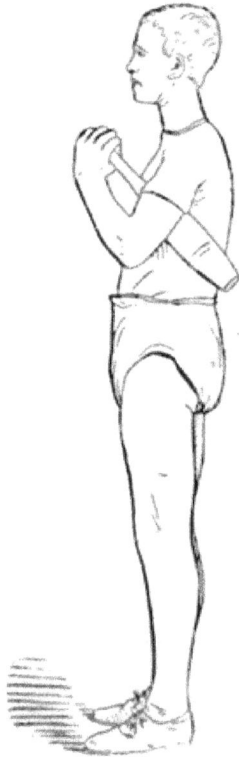

Fig. 154.

Fig. 154 illustrates a "catch" or finish.

SECOND SERIES.   WALTZ   OR   MARCH TIME.

(Waltz time perferable.) For position, see Fig. 138.

1. Double heart-shaped circle out 4 times, reverse 4 times (Fig. 153 shows method of passing the hands).

2. Short shoulder-circle out with the right club; at the same time make a heart-shaped circle out with the left hand 2 times.

3. Same as No. 2, but left hand makes short circle, right hand makes heart-shaped circle. (Repeat exercises Nos. 2 and 3.)

4. Take the reel 8 counts (Fig. 143).

5. A *drop* circle twice on each (Fig. 149). *Raise* circle twice on each side (Fig. 150). *Inside* drop twice on each side (Fig. 155). *Parallel circle* once on the right, once on the left (Fig. 151), once more on the right, then a complete pendulum from left to right, and bring the clubs to position.

6. Make a "6-circle parallel,"—that is, a double short circle to the right,—one shoulder-high, one elbow-high, one double lower front, one raise circle elbow-high on the left, one shoulder-high on the left, and one double back shoulder-circle.

7. Make a "7-circle parallel," same as 6-circle parallel with this exception: there is one extra circle made on the right.

8. Make a *drop* circle on the right, a *raise* circle on the left, an *inside* drop on the right, a *parallel* circle on the left, a *drop* on the right; from this swing to a reel, which is taken 4 times.

9. A reel and lower front combination 4 times. This is made by making two short shoulder-circles out with the right hand, while the left hand makes the lower front.

10. Double short shoulder-circles to the front, out, and inside the arm, and catch the clubs on the 8th count (Fig. 154).

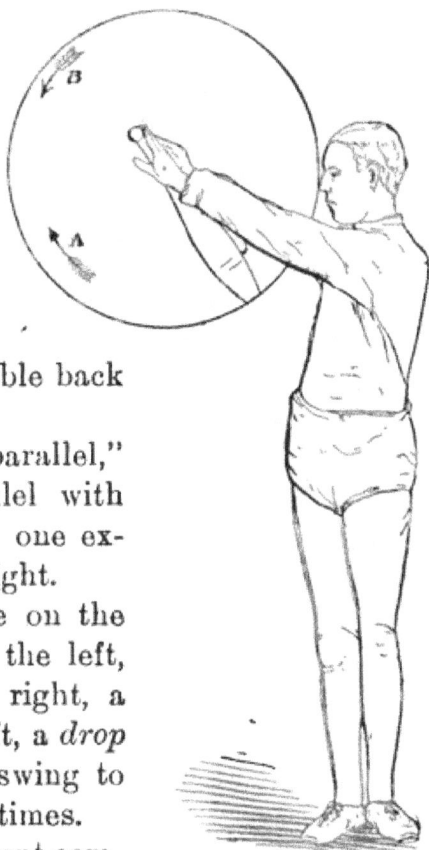

FIG. 155.

FIG. 155.—An inside raise The clubs are held nearly parallel to the floor. The points or ends are raised,, and pass inside of the arm following the arrow *A*. If the clubs follow the arrow *B*, an inside drop would be made.

THIRD SERIES.   WALTZ TIME.

Position, see Fig. **138.**

1. Reel; 4 times.

2. Reel and lower front ; 4 times.

3. **Reel and high side circles.** This is the same as the 2d exercise, with the exception that, instead of making the **lower front circle, the** club swings up and the circle is made on the opposite side of the body, shoulder-high.

4. Reel and **combination of one lower front, one** circle elbow-high on **left, and one** shoulder-high on the left. While the right hand is making these three circles in front of the body, the left hand makes three *shoulder* circles to the left. This combination is made 3 times ; on the 4th count, make one drop circle on the left ; and from this swing to the double overhead parallel (Fig. **148**), which is taken 7 times ; on the 8th count, come to position.

5. Short reel, same **as No. 1,** but the hands do not go lower than the shoulders. (See Fig. **139.**) Position on the 8th count.

6. Make a half outside drop, a half inside drop, one full outside drop, pendulum, and same on the left ; 4 times.

7. From the left side swing across to the right side and begin the double parallel circles across the front of the body, first with the right and then with the left. (See Fig. 152.) On the 8th count come to position.

8. Double lower back and reverse ; 4 times (Fig. 142).

9. Double lower back combined with double lower front, from right to left and from left to right ; 4 times.

10. "The Divide."—The left club makes a lower front, while the right club makes a lower back ; without stopping, make a lower back with the left hand and a lower front with the right hand, and swing the clubs up to the left side shoulder-high. Reverse this exercise. Take 4 times.

CHAPTER XI.

THESE are made with light pine poles from 8 to 12 feet in length and from one to one and a quarter inches in diameter. They can be easily made by a carpenter and at a small cost. It is not even necessary that the poles be round. If they are square with the corners rounded enough to prevent the wood cutting the hands it will be sufficient. Long brush poles can be purchased at hardware stores at from 10 to 20 cents apiece. For exhibition work these poles can be covered with silesia of different colors, or they can be adorned with ribbons. The author does not recommend this exercise for large classes unless the teacher is a first-class disciplinarian. To make the work a success, it is necessary the scholars be of nearly the same height. The poles may be suspended along the sides of the room 2 to 3 feet from the floor. When the time comes for this exercise the class is formed into 1 or 2 long lines; they are then marched to their different positions on the floor, the shorter members of the class being at the head of the lines, which stand from front to back and which are made up of from 8 to 12 pupils. After the various lines are formed, the monitors, who have been specially drilled for this purpose, bring and place the

164

poles alongside of the lines, one on the right and one
on the left, about 6 inches from the feet.   At a chord
the pupils stoop down, grasp the poles and come
back to position.   The first time the exercise is taken
the poles can be placed on the floor and in position
before the motions are begun.   It will then be much
easier for the different files to march to their places,

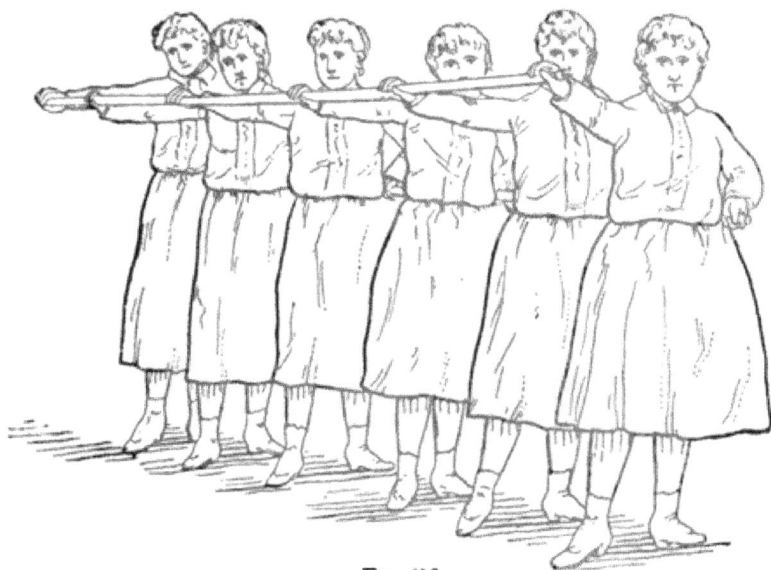

Fig. 156.
Pole shoulder-high to the right, stepping motion with the right foot.

but after this it will be better for the poles to be han-
dled by monitors.   The exercises are taken to waltz
time.

I. *Step* right foot to the right and swing pole
shoulder-high to the right 8 times, same on left side.
(Fig. 156.)

II. On count 1, raise and lower the body on the toes ;

count 2, swing the poles up and lower to side ; 16 counts (Fig. 157).

III. Raise the right pole OUT; from this position swing pole to the front, swing back to first position, pole DOWN; this will take 4 counts. Take the same exercise on the left side.

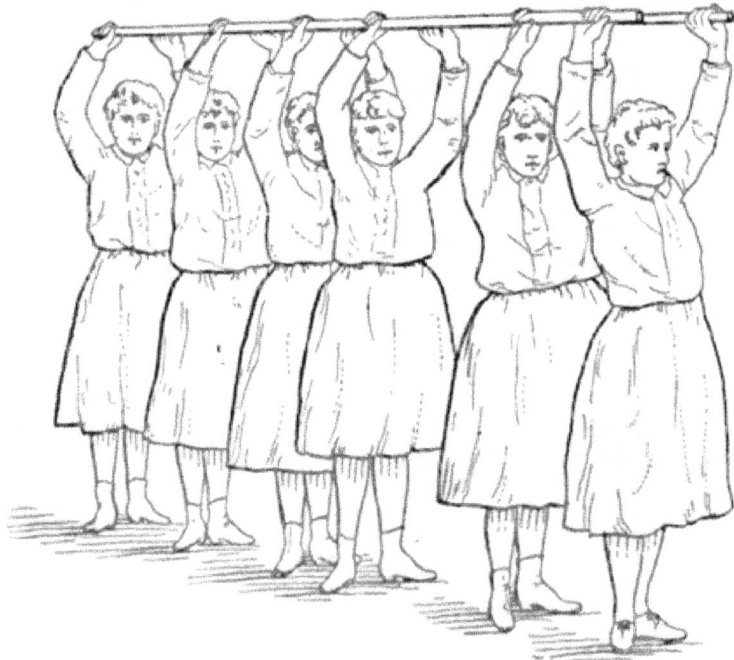

FIG. 157.—Poles up.

A stepping motion of the right foot to the right, from there to the front, from there to the right again, and heels together, can be combined with the arm motion.

IV. Take the arm motions with both arms as in No. III.

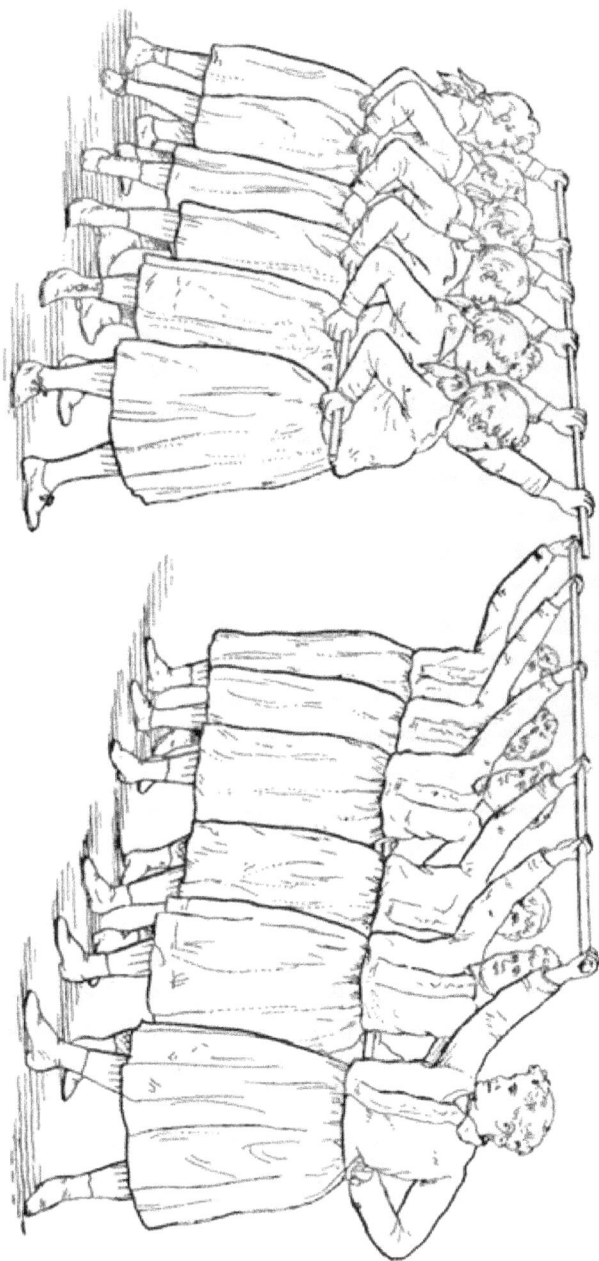

Fig. 158.
Lines charging towards each other.

V. **Left hand** on the hip, charge to the right, the right hand up; same to the left; 8 times. If in **this** exercise there is an even number on lines, **then have two** lines charge towards each other for 4 counts, and away from each other for 4 counts (Fig. 158).

VI. Count 1, take position **as in** exercise I; 2, charge the right foot diagonally back, swing right hand diag-

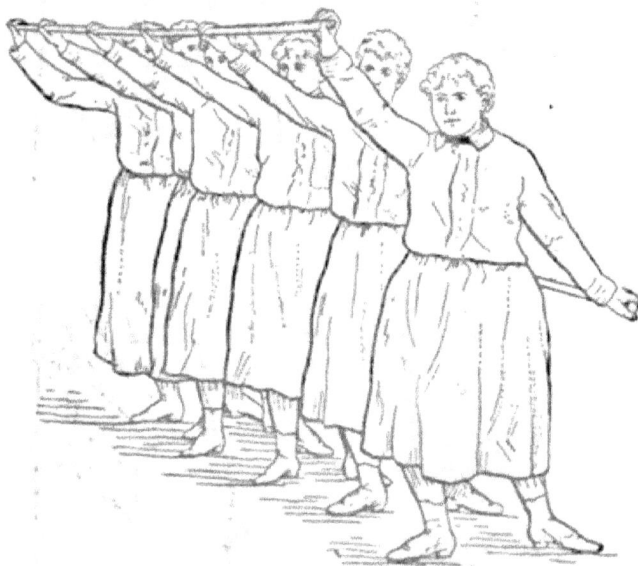

Fig. 159.
Swaying motion to the right.

onally back shoulder-high, **look in** the same direction; 3, come back to position 1; 4, hands DOWN, heels together.

VII. Charge right foot to the right, raise right hand diagonally out and up, left hand hip-high to the left (Fig. 159); now sway the body from right to left, at the same time lowering the right and raising the left hand.

Sway body from right to left for 7 counts, coming to position on 8. Take the same exercise on the left side.

VIII. The two lines charge away from each other as in exercise V. This position they hold for 8 counts, then the two lines turn on the balls of both feet, kneel

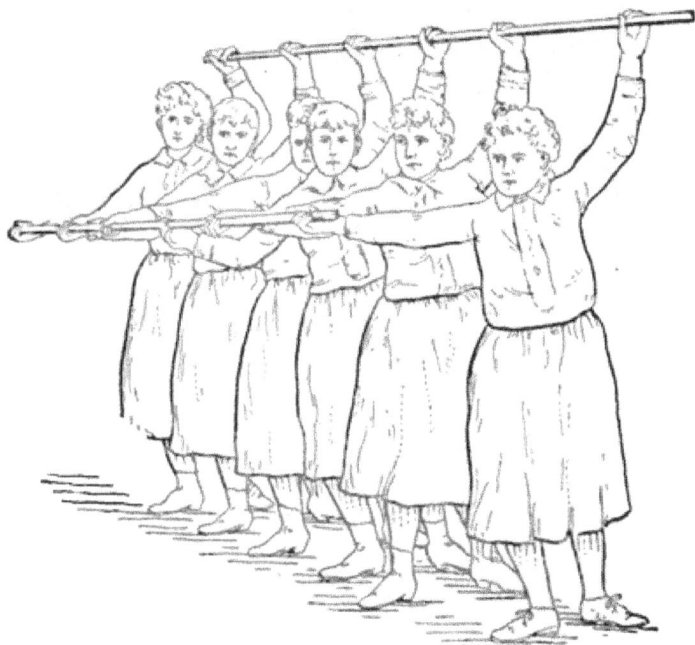

FIG. 160.
Right-angle charge to the right.

and touch the outside knee to the floor, outside hand on the hip, inside arm up, face slightly raised (Fig. 161).

The poles can be brought to the shoulders; and by changing the position of the hands, or the "hold," many motions, such as charging, right angles (Fig. 160), thrusting, swinging, etc., can be taken from this position. A line of pupils can work with a single pole, grasping it with both hands, in which case many of the exercises already described can be given. The teacher must not forget the difference between a "line" and a "file" of pupils.

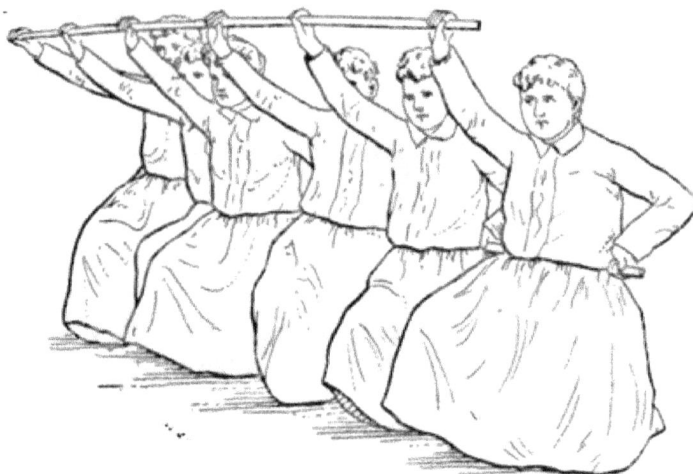

FIG. 161.
A simple posture.

Fig. 161 represents the pupils on the left in Fig. 158 if they execute the maneuver described in VIII.

CHAPTER XII.

THE short sticks used for the three series with the wands will do for these fencing exercises. In this as in other maneuvers the work is arranged for pupils, and will not therefore conform to the rules that may govern any particular system of fencing.

Pupils should be taught the position of "on guard" first without holding the stick or sword. From the position of attention pupils *left oblique face*, or half face to the left, and turn the feet to an angle of 90 instead of 60 degrees; thus forming a right angle, the right foot pointing to the front and the left foot to the left.

Rest the back of the left hand on the hip (see Fig. 162), lower the body about six inches by bending both knees, but keep the heels together. Slide the right foot front twice its length, the feet preserving their angle of 90 degrees. Both feet are on the same line, or if the boards of the floor run from front to rear both heels are on the same board. Both knees are bent. The weight of the body rests more on the left

171

than on the right leg. Raise the right arm, nearly half bent, to the front until the hand is chest-high, palm of the hand up (Fig. 162). Face front.

The fact has been emphasized that the right foot points front and the right arm is to the front. This

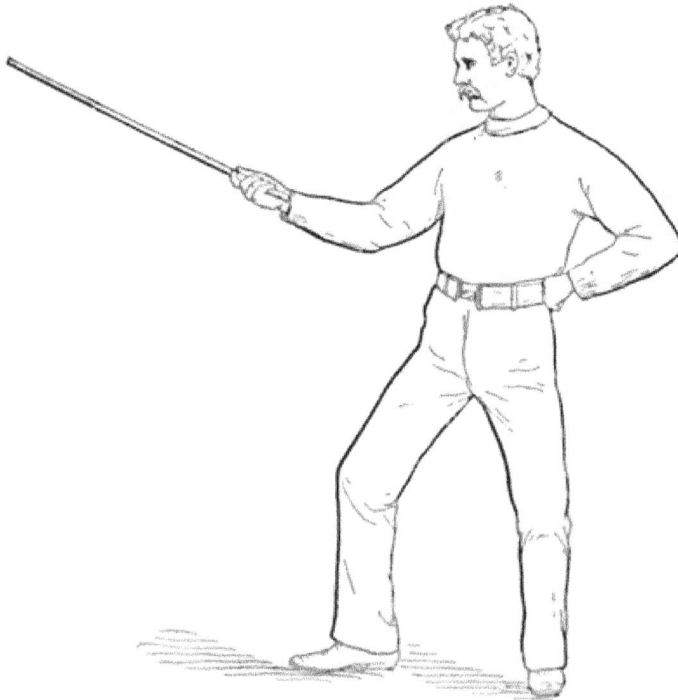

FIG. 162.
On guard.

is done because the shoulders are at a left oblique, and the inclination is to point the sword in the same direction. By referring to the figure the correct position of "on guard" will be seen.

Teach pupils to take the position in several movements as described, then direct them to take it in one
movement. When this is learned give them the sword.
This is first held at "carry arms" or, better, "carry

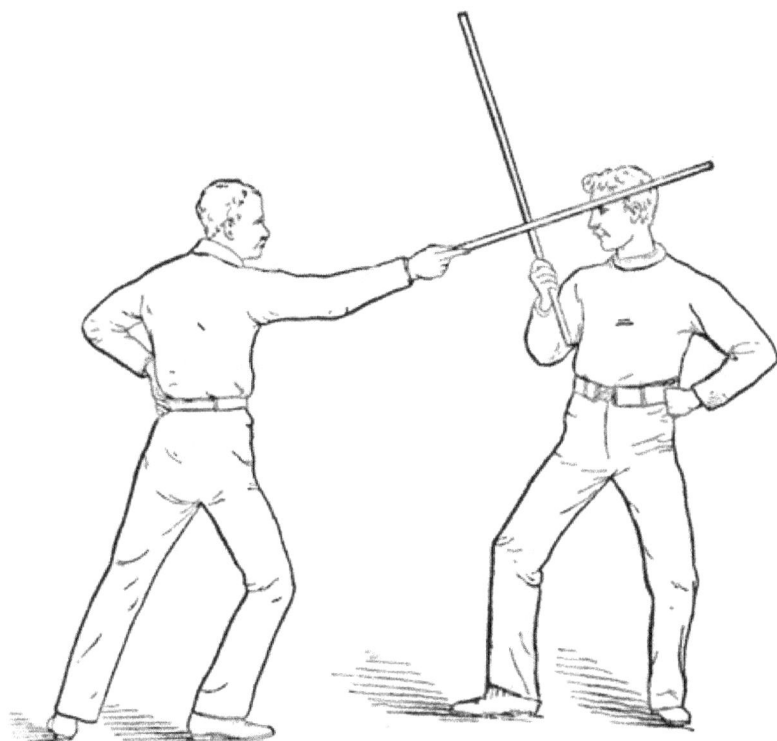

FIG. 163.
Left cheek blow and guard.

swords." When in position the sword points to the
front (not left oblique). The point of the sword is
at the height of the eye.

Teachers will find that younger pupils and girls can-

not hold the position seen in Fig. 162, as it soon
fatigues them.   They can hold a **position** similar **to**
that of **" charge** bayonets" with the right **foot front,**
right **knee** slightly bent, left leg
back and straight.   After pupils

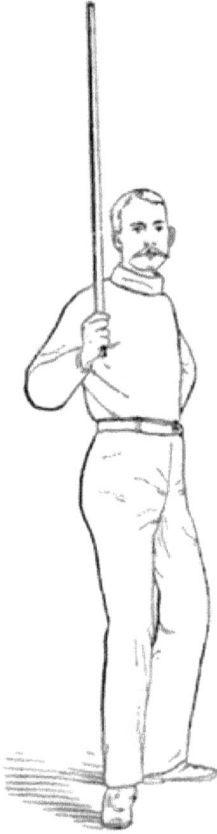

Fig. 164.

Right cheek guard.

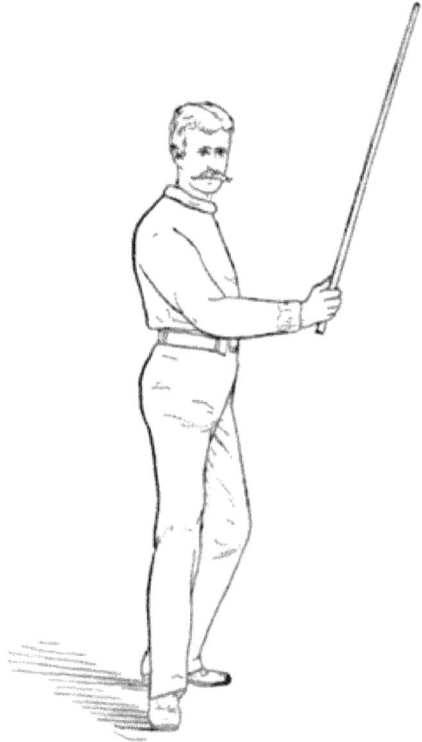

Fig. 165.

Left shoulder guard.

have mastered the position, drill them in "swaying."
They are now ready for the blows and guards.

There are seven of each :

1. **Head** Guard.—The sword is held parallel to the floor, 8 inches above and in front of the head.

2. **Left** Cheek Guard.—Right hand shoulder-high on the left. Sword perpendicular, but in front as well as to the left of the face. (See right-hand figure, No. 163.)

3. **Right Cheek Guard.**—Right hand shoulder-high to the front, sword perpendicular, but to the front as well as to the right of the face (Fig. 164).

4. **Left Shoulder Guard.**—Same as left cheek, but the hand is held to the left a little higher than the elbow. The left shoulder is thrown well back in this guard (Fig. 165).

5. **Right Shoulder Guard.**—Same as right cheek, but the hand is elbow-high to the front and right of the shoulder (Fig. 166).

6. **Left Lower Guard.**—Swing the sword down across the right knee and over to the left side ; the hand is hip-high, thumb to the front. The point of the sword is down.

The sword to the left as well as to the front of the left thigh.

7. **Right Lower Guard.**—Same as on the left, but the sword is to the right and front of the right thigh. The back of the hand is front (Fig. 167).

Blows.—If two pupils are facing each other, and in position, the—

1st blow will be aimed at the top of the head ;

2d, at the left cheek ;

3d, at the right cheek ;

4th, at the left shoulder ;

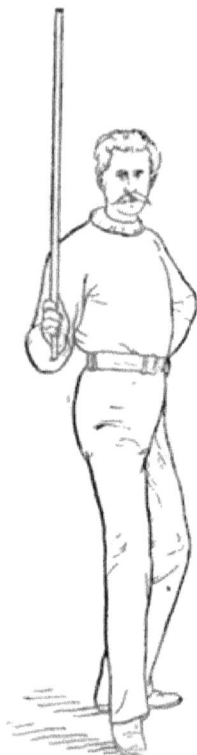

FIG. 166.
Right shoulder
guard.

5th, at the right shoulder;

6th, at the middle of the left thigh;

7th, at the middle of the right thigh.

These blows are warded off by a guard of the corresponding number.

When striking a blow, sway forward; then come back to the position, the sword always on the right.

When guarding, keep the body still, using only the arm. After the pupils have been thoroughly drilled in the position and guards, they are then formed in "twos."

At the command "Take your distance," they step away from and face each other. Each pupil places the point of his sword against the waist of his neighbor and the handle against his own waist.

The sword is held in the right hand, the left arm is at the side. Heels together.

At command "Take your position," the pupils take the position of "on guard" (Fig. 162), swords crossed.

For practice, let No. 1 give the head blow 8 times, while No. 2 guards; between the blows, come to position, clicking the swords lightly. Next, No. 2

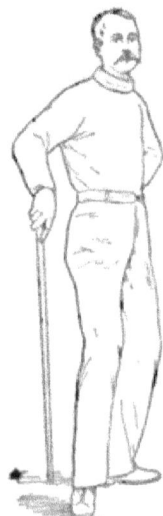

FIG. 167.
Right lower
guard.

strikes while No. 1 guards. **And in the same manner** teach the various blows. It will be more difficult to teach blows **6 and 7** than the others.

After pupils **have** learned to give each blow 8 times, they can **give** four, then two blows, and finally one.

The **exercise can also** be given **without coming** to position **each time.**

The one **who** guards can also strike immediately at his opponent. This is done in Lunging.

Lunging. — From on guard, **No. 1 lunges** forward and gives **a blow.** No. 2 steps the **right**

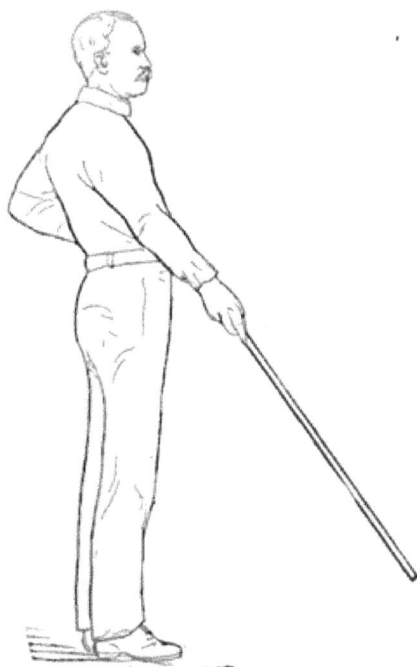

Fig 168.
Lowering the sword.

foot back of the **left, and** guards. **Without coming** to position, No. 2 **will** lunge and No. 1 **will step back.** Seven blows can be given in this manner.

By referring to Fig. **173, a correct** idea **can be had** of the lunge and guard.

It is **not expected** that **girls will** take a full lunge **while** in ordinary costume.

This arrangement of fencing is more like the broadsword than the foil exercise. **All thrusting motions** should be avoided.   A little care on the teacher's part will prevent accidents.

Salutes.—A short salute to the opponent at the beginning and end of the "bout" is described.

1. Form Twos. — Half face to the left and lower the sword. The half face has been described. To lower the sword, which is at "carry," drop the point down until the sword and arm are in the same line. The hand is hip-high to the front, arm rigid. (See Fig. 168.)

2. Elevate the sword. Swing the point of the sword up to the front until the sword and arm are in the same line, the hand a little higher than the head.   (See Fig. 169.)

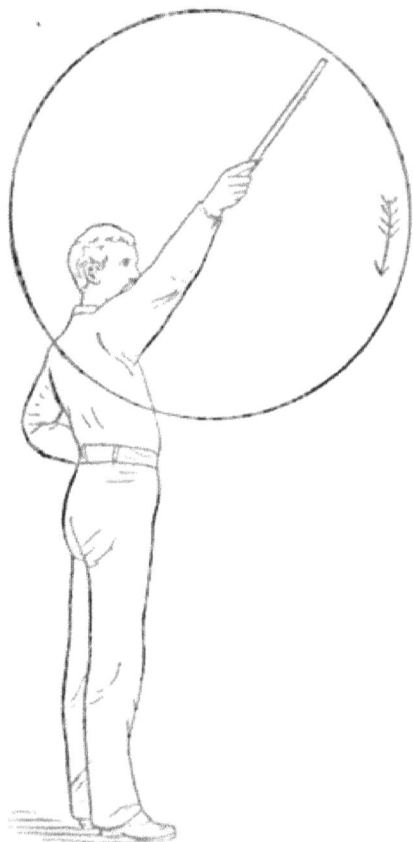

FIG. 169.
Elevate the sword.

3. Pass to a Guard.   From an "elevate" bring the sword down in front, both arms slightly curved.   The back of the left hand may be above the stick, which rests between the knuckles of the second and third fingers (see Fig. 170), or it may be grasped by the

left hand as when DOWN. Now raise the sword up as in Fig. 171, and from this position come to "on guard." (See Fig. 162.)

4. Pass to a Salute. Proceed as in "passing to a guard" until the sword is up. Then bring the sword to the position seen in

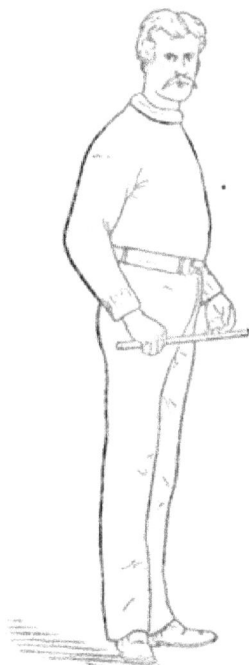

FIG. 170.
Sword down.

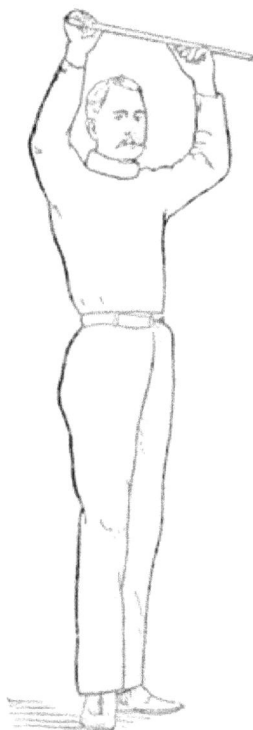

FIG. 171.
Sword up.

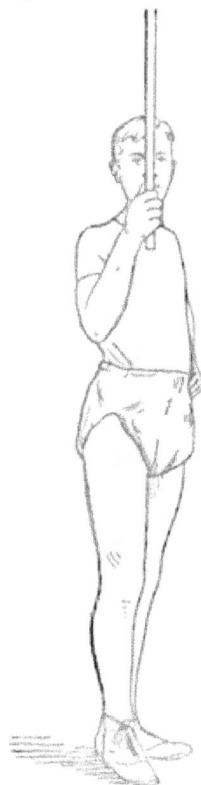

FIG. 172.
Face salute.

Fig. 172. Now swing the sword down to the right, next back to the position in Fig. 172; from here either assume "on guard" or "carry arms." These maneuvers can be done to march, waltz, or polka time.

A Regular Series.

We shall deal only with a "two." The pupil on the right is No. 1. The pupil on the left is No. 2. Swords at "carry arms." At a chord, "Take distance."

With the beginning of the music.—

Swords down, **4 counts** (Fig. **170**);

Swords up, 4 counts (Fig. 171);

Lower swords, **4 counts** (Fig. 168);

Elevate **swords**, 4 counts (Fig. 169);

On guard, **but cross** swords below **on the left side, 4** counts;

Cross swords below on the **right side, 4 counts**;

Cross swords above (position for fencing), **4** counts;

Heels together and " face salute," **1 count** (Fig. 172);

Swing sword down to right, **1 count**;

Face salute, 1 count;

"On guard," 1 count **(Fig. 162)**.

The **last** four movements **are** quickly made, as but one count is allowed for each.

This finishes **the short** salute to partners, and **leaves** both pupils on guard ready for fencing. No. **1 strikes** the first blow 2 times. Then No. **2 does the** same. In a like manner the seven blows are given, swords coming to position between each **blow. This** makes a round of two blows each.

Next, **No. 1** strikes the first blow once, and No. 2 does the same. Continue through the seven blows in a similar manner. This is a round of one blow each.

Repeat the round of one blow. The striking exercises so far have taken **7** measures of music of **16** counts each.

Lunges.—Do not come to position between the lunges. No. 1 lunges and strikes the head blow; he holds this position for 4 counts. Then No. 2 gives the head blow, and holds the position for 4 counts. In this way proceed with 5 blows, omitting those at the

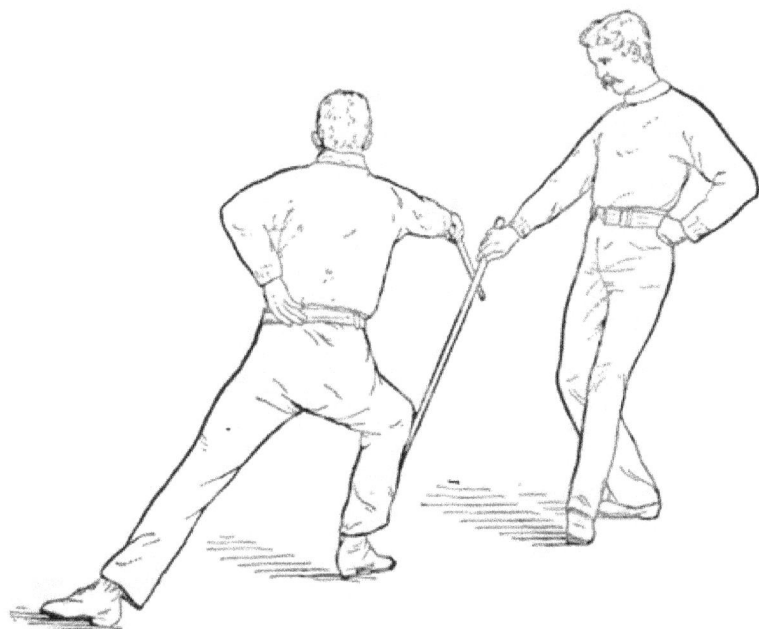

FIG. 173.
Right lower guard and step back. In this cut the left-hand figure lunges.

cheek. The last lunge will be made by No. 2, the strike and guard being at the right thigh, after which there will be left but 8 counts to finish a measure of music (Fig. 173).

On two counts, the pupils front face and come to a position of face salute (Fig. 172). To do this, No. 1 steps forward, and turns to the front on his left heel.

No. 2 steps back, and turns to the front on his left heel. Swing sword down to the right side, 2 counts; carry swords, 2 counts. Pupils step side by side 2

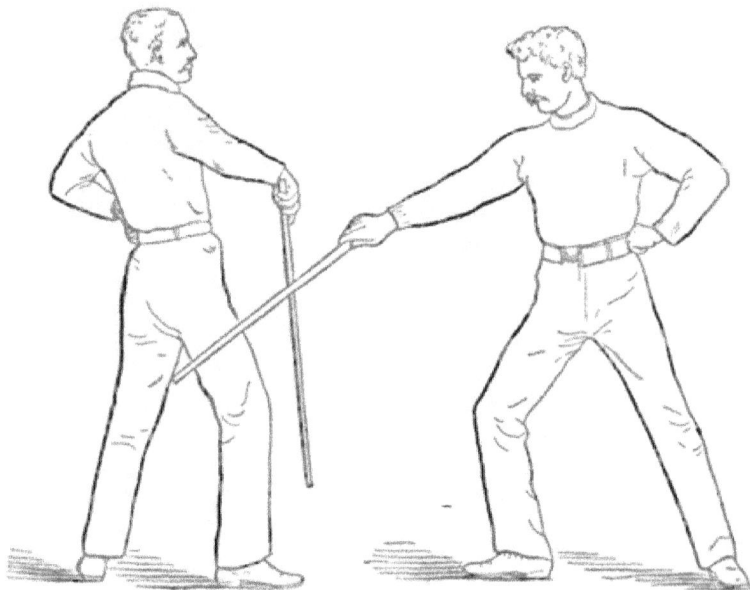

Fig. 174.
Right lower blow and guard.

counts; from which position they can march from the room or to their seats.

The Brooklyn Bridge March goes well to the fencing exercise. (See p. 234.)

CHAPTER XIII.

THESE positions can be given to boys and young men. They should be held for 8 or 16 counts.

A very pleasing effect can be had if several well-built young men will dress in full white tights, wear white wigs, and powder their faces; then take these positions under a calcium light.

The background should be black: it can be made of black calico or silesia. A curtain should be drawn before each change. For additional postures, the teacher is referred to any work on statuary, where may be found, among others,—

Apollo Belvedere,
Discobolus (2),
Athlete (2),
Boxer (2),
Gladiator (2),
The following are good: Boxer No. 1. (See Fig. 175.)

Boxer No. 2. (See Fig. 176.)
Putting the Shot, first position. (See Fig. 177.)
Putting the Shot, second position. (See Fig. 178.)
The Gladiator. (See Fig. 179.)
The Start. (See Fig. 180.)
At Rest. (See Fig. 181.)

183

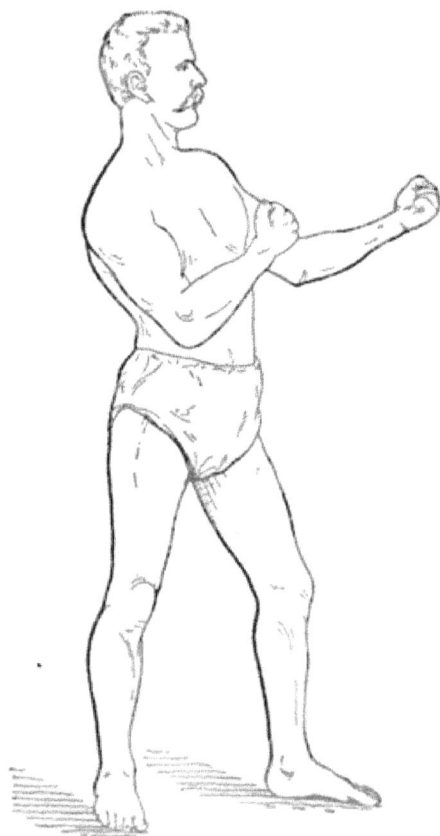

Fig. 175.
The boxer on guard.

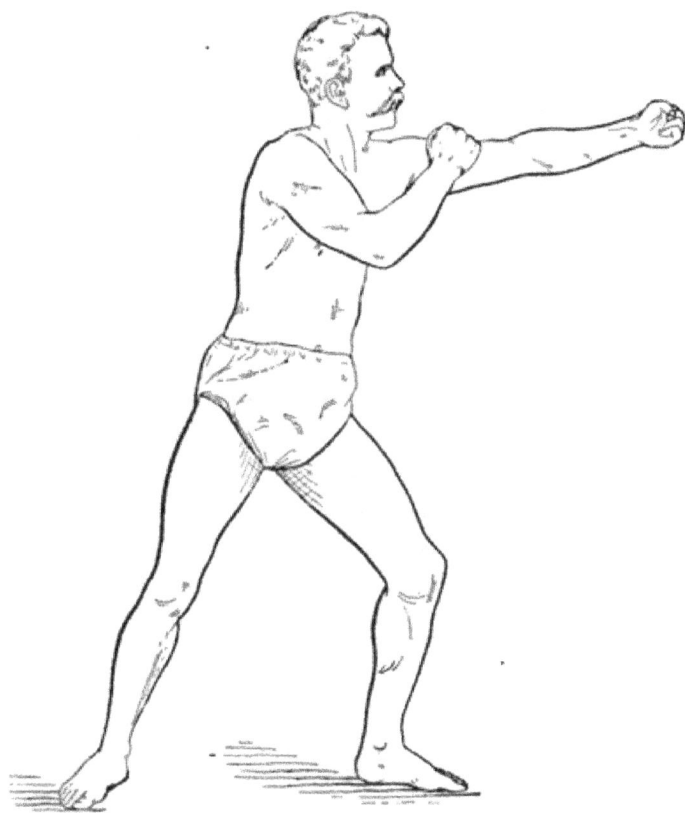

FIG. 176.
The boxer left-hand lead.

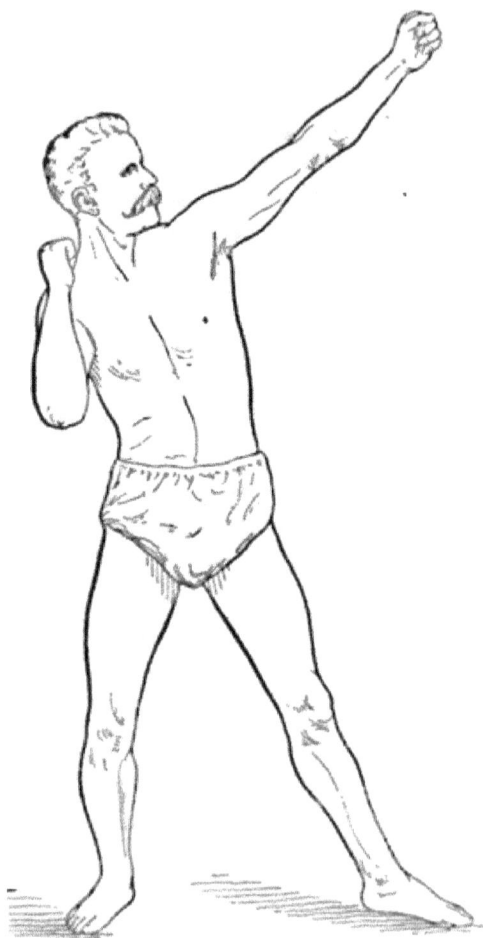

FIG. 177.
Putting the shot; the start.

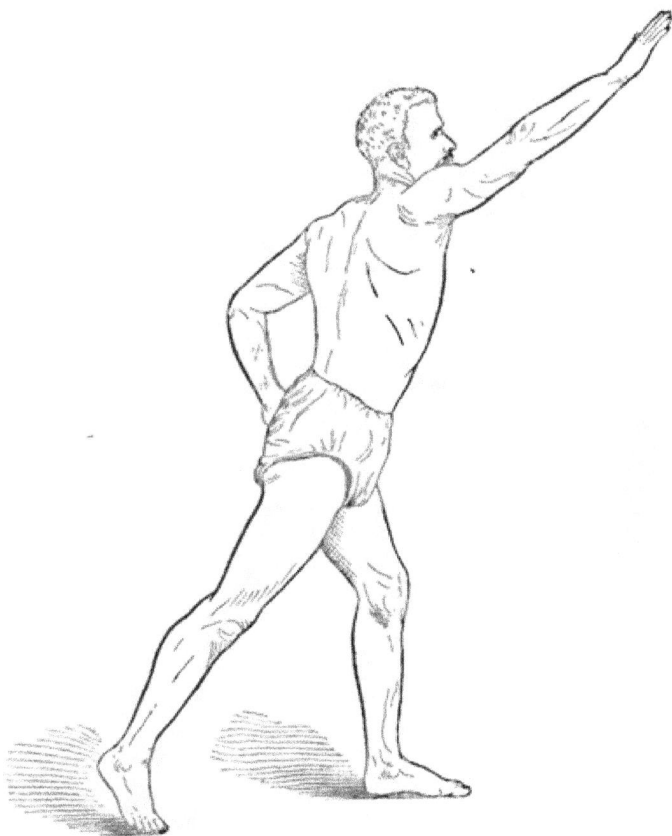

Fig. 178.
Putting the shot; the finish.

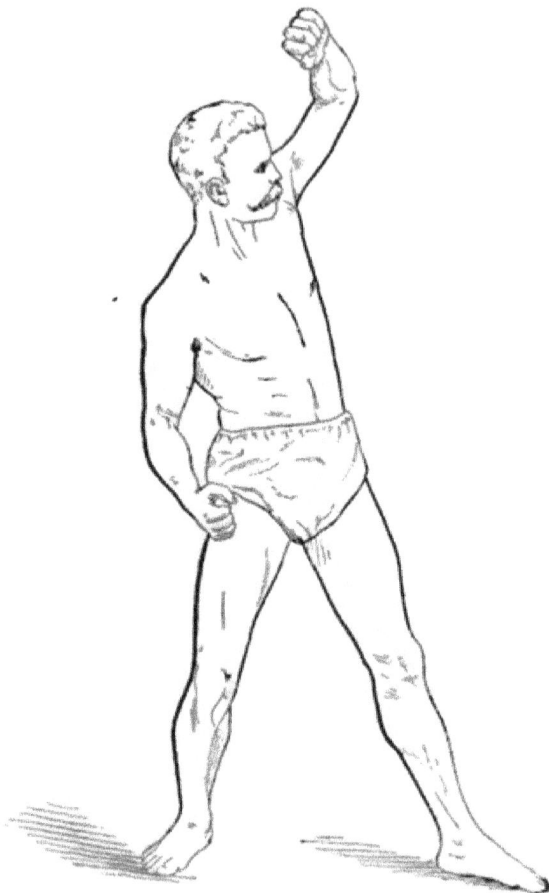

FIG. 179.
The gladiator.

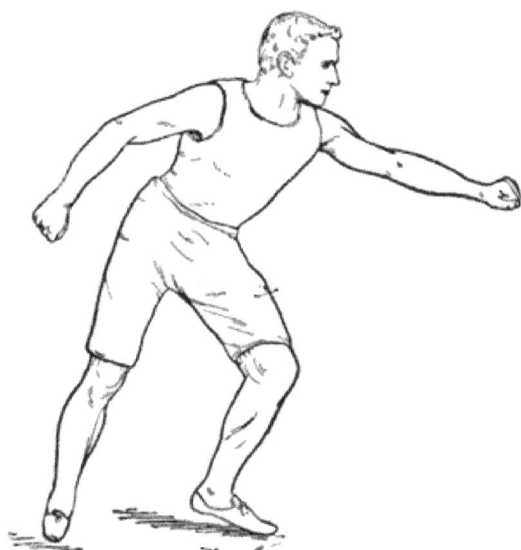

FIG. 180.
The start.

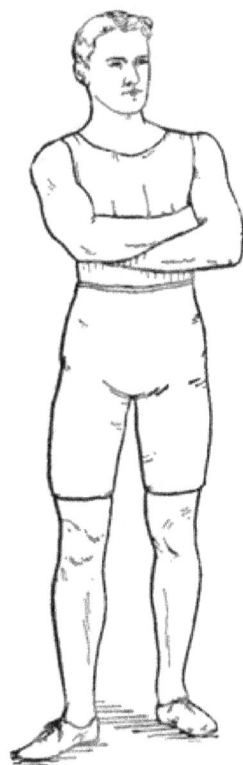

FIG. 181.
At rest.

SIMPLE ATTITUDES.

The following attitudes are given, not to express any emotion or feeling, but merely for nerve-training. They should be accompanied by some pretty ballad music

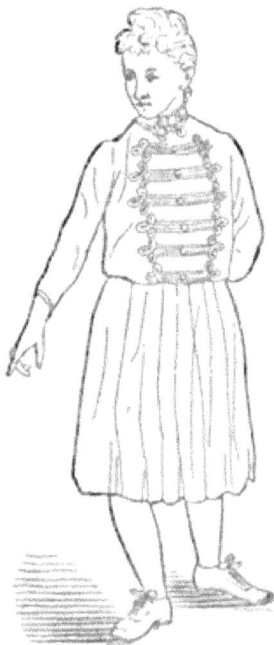

Fig. 183.

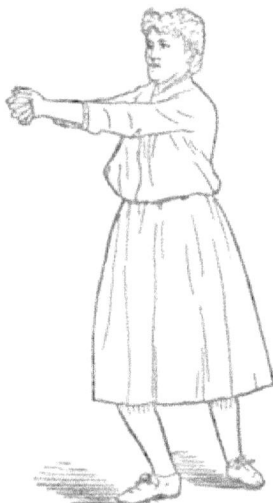

Fig. 182.

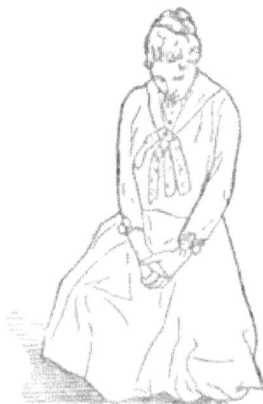

Fig. 184.

softly played. They will do well as a finish for any exercise in free gymnastics.

Each position is held for 8 counts. The primary or starting position should be with the hands clasped

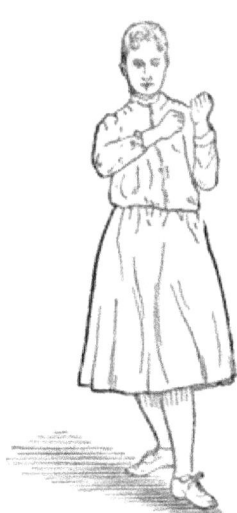

FIG. 185.

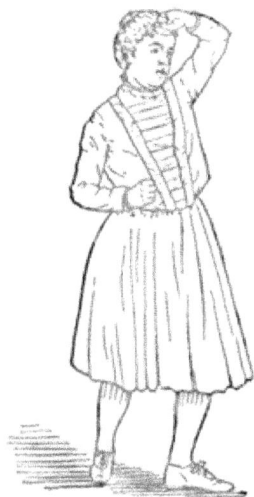

FIG. 186.

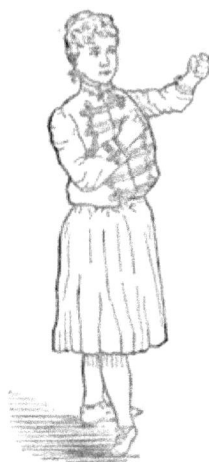

FIG. 187.

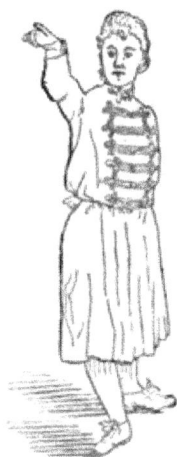

FIG. 188.

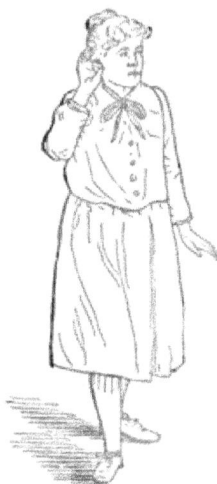

FIG. 190.

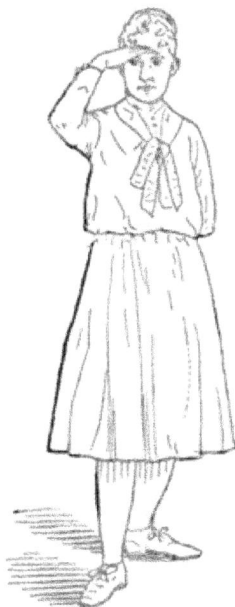

FIG. 189.

in front or with arms folded, the pupil at rest. From the starting position the posture No. 182 is taken. This is held for 8 counts.

Without coming back to rest, the pupil passes to the attitude seen in Fig. 183. This position is held for 8 counts.

From this the pupil will assume the posture seen in Fig. 184, from which she comes to the position of rest, which is held for 8 counts.

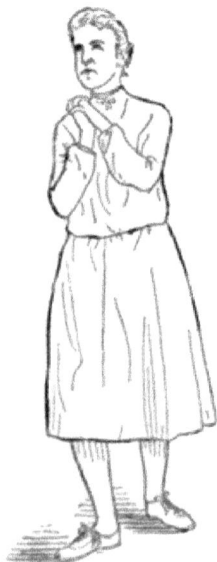

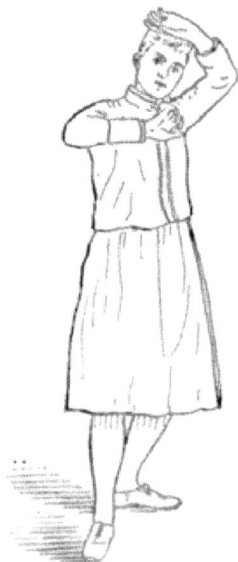

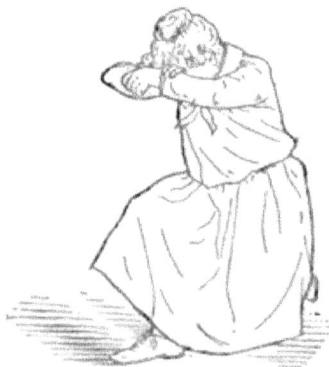

Fig. 191.   Fig. 192.   Fig. 193.

It will be seen that we have taken for these four positions 32 counts.

The same work should be done on the left side.

The **first** group of simple attitudes is made up of Figs. 182, 183, and 184.

The second group is **made up of** Figs. 185, 186, and **187.**

The third group is composed of Figs. 188, 189, 190.
The fourth group includes Figs. 191, 192, and 193.

Each group is taken on both the right and the left sides, and each one requires 64 counts. In teaching these attitudes, do not hurry. Drill the pupil well in the position of the arms, legs, head, and general position.

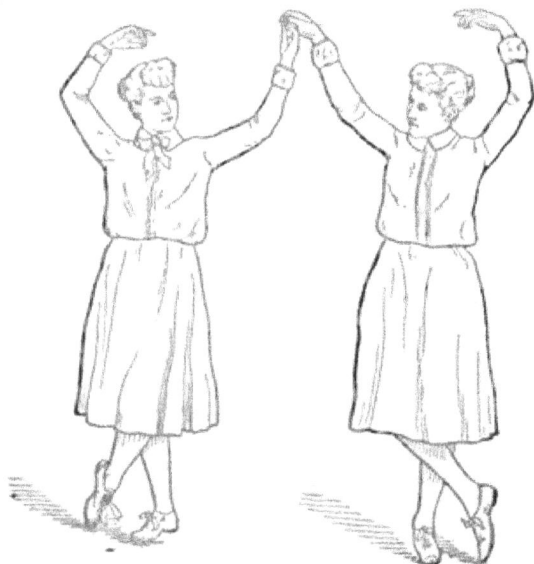

FIG. 194.

By teaching the attitudes in sections, the result is more satisfactory. Not more than two positions should be given at one lesson. An interesting exhibition can be given if the teacher will illustrate some poem, which is first read aloud, by the postures which the poem suggests. A large number of positions can be learned if the different passions are expressed, or if statues and pictures are illustrated. The melodies from "Mother Goose" can thus be used.

CHAPTER **XIV.**

AT every lesson there should be breathing exercises of some kind.

Children do **not** readily **see** the difference **between** intercostal, diaphragmatic, abdominal, and **other kinds** of breathing. Direct them to take a deep, **full breath, and they** will do what **you** want **better than when you try to** explain the difference between **the styles named. Try these** methods :

1. Children **mark time** or **march, and hold** their breath **5, 10,** or 20 steps, **and so** on.

2. Sighing and hissing for **5, 10, or** 20 counts.

3. Inhaling for a certain number of counts.

4. Whistling.

5. Running.

6. Fill the lungs full, raise the elbows, **arms** flexed ; then force them down and back a **few** times.

7. Counting aloud while exercising.

8. Pronouncing the vowels.

9. Spelling slowly.

10. Pronouncing the vowels aspirated, with explosive force.—" Ha! Ha!" etc.

194

CHAPTER XV.

MEASUREMENTS.

TEACHERS of gymnastics should strive to convince people of the importance of physical education. They should offer a quality of work, the results of which will persuade the most skeptical parents and pupils to their belief. They should teach that many of the deformities or defects caused by failure to exercise can be remedied by gymnastics. They should try to prove that the nearest approach to a perfect physique in a boy or girl is through a system of careful training. Moreover, they should take steps to ascertain just what constitutes a perfect physique, or what the proportions of a well-built boy or girl are. The surest way to do this is for the teacher to thoroughly understand his work, to be posted on the current literature pertaining to physical education, and, above all, to believe thoroughly in this subject. The teacher should adopt any honest method of winning the confidence of the children and, through the children, the parents.

A feasible plan is to adopt some system of examinations or measurements of the children, and to use simple physical tests. Little has been done about the measurements of school children in this country; consequently there is not much to say about them that is positive. It is hoped that **all teachers of** gymnastics **who handle** school **children will spare time** enough to take their **age, height, weight, and lung capacity, and to** notice the result **of** exercise upon the defects that have been mentioned, that something definite may be reached. **If** teachers will, **in** addition to the items mentioned, take a few girth, width, **and length** measurements, **their** statistics will be far more valuable. Too much importance cannot be attached to the accuracy **of** any test or measurement. The **temptation** to exaggerate to prove a certain end **is** strong, but it should be overcome. Be honest in taking measurements; and if your figures **are not as satisfactory as** you hoped they would be, **don't add a little.** Accept the situation as it **is. We** are striving **to** prove the necessity **of** gymnastic **drill; and nothing** will hasten this quicker than honesty.

In this short chapter **on** measurements, we shall give a few figures that may serve for comparison.

These statistics are taken from some of the largest private schools in this country. They represent **the** measurements of several thousand pupils **of the ages** given, and they extend over a period of five **years.**

It must be taken into consideration that the pupils whose measurements **are** given not only take drill in the gymnasium, but they are from families who can offer everything in the shape of social and hygienic surroundings. These two facts of course carry weight: all of the children in the public schools do not enjoy these privileges; there will consequently be a difference in the height and weight in favor of the pupils in the private school. In addition to the statistics from the schools mentioned, there are a large number of measurements taken from the public schools in Boston. (See Dr. Bowditch's valuable Report to the Massachusetts Board of Health, 1877.)

The figures given have been carefully examined by expert accountants. For the benefit of those who wish to go deeper in the subject, the rules for physical measurements and examination proposed by the American Association for the Advancement of Physical Education are given. They are the best and most reliable.

Teachers can interest their pupils by giving them a few simple strength tests once or twice a year. In some public and even private schools it is not always convenient or popular to take many measurements; but if only a few records are kept, and the teacher will take some interest in them, there will be, as a result, an increase in the interest of the pupil. We give in this chapter the diagram of a blank to be used in the measurement of school children (Fig. 195).

Fig. 196 shows the average height and weight given by Dr. Bowditch, of Boston, for the public-school children of that city between the ages of 5 and 8 years, taken without shoes; otherwise the ordinary clothing is worn when these measurements are taken. The weight of clothing is about 8 pounds for boys and 7 for girls. We have also given the average height, weight, and lung capacity of pupils in prominent private schools in and near New York City. These figures are given for comparison. A chart has been planned by Dr. J. W.

DEPARTMENT OF PHYSICAL EDUCATION

OF THE

ADELPHI ACADEMY, BROOKLYN, N. Y.

PHYSICAL **CONDITION OF**

GRADE

DATE.	Age.	Height.	Weight.	Lung Capacity.	What it should be.				

AGE	6.	7.	8.	9.	10.	11.	12.	13.	14.	15.	
Height..	46.40	48.90	50.17	52.26	54.43	56.86	57.79	59.92	62.53	64.38	BOYS.
Weight .	47.55	56.44	58.09	63.86	71.42	76.17	81.81	95.20	105.15	113.81	
Lung Capacity	64	80	88	106	124	144	150	168	188	205	
Height..	46.11	47.95	49.82	52.03	53.99	57.06	59.17	60.89	63.38	68.12	GIRLS.
Weight .	46.55	50.83	56.37	62.32	71.52	80.81	90.08	99.61	108.99	112.80	
Lung Capacity	35	40	48	65	80	106	125	136	155	150	

[The above figures show the average height, weight, and about the lung capacity of the pupils in a number of the private schools in and near Brooklyn. They are given only for comparison. It cannot be said **of** them that they indicate just what the averages should be.]

Parents are earnestly requested to notify the Physician in charge of this department, of Physical Defects, if any, that exist in their children, that he may regulate the exercises accordingly.

                                        Director Physical Education.

FIG. 195.— A simple chart to be used in schools

Seaver, of **Yale College.** It represents the measurements of **thousands of American** college-students, arranged according to age. It does not **follow** strictly the order of measurements **given by the** special committee, page 201.

For details concerning this compilation of **figures,** the reader is referred to **Dr.** Seaver, Yale **College,** New Haven, Conn.

Dr. **Edward** Hitchcock, director of the Pratt Gymnasium, at Amherst College, has arranged his anthropometric *data* in book form. It contains the result of many **years of** hard **work, and** is a **most valuable** compilation.

The **author is** under obligations **to Dr.** Hitchcock for the valuable suggestions he has generously given.

The simple chart (Fig. 195) would not do so well **for public** schools; as the average height, weight, **and lung** capacity of public school children are not **so large as** those taken **from the** best private schools.

A wealthier **class of pupils** attend private institutions. The hygienic surroundings are better, **and the** smaller number of **pupils warrants** better **care than is found** in the **public** schools. This will account **for** the difference **that** may be **seen when** comparing the *data* obtained from the two **sources.**

On **page 200** will be found **statistics taken from Dr.** Bowditch's report on the growth of children **(Fig. 196).** They represent the **height and weight of thousands of** public-school children **in Boston.**

AGE	6.	7.	8.	9.	10.	11.	12.	13.	14.	15.	
Height..	43.75	45.74	47.76	49.69	51.68	53.33	55.11	57.21	59.88	62.30	Boys.
Weight..	45.17	49.07	53.92	59.23	65.30	70.18	76.92	84.84	94.91	107.10	
Height..	43.35	45.52	47.58	49.37	51.34	53.42	55.88	58.16	59.94	61.10	Girls.
Weight..	43.28	47.46	52.04	57.07	62.35	68.84	78.31	88.65	98.43	106.08	

F ɪ ɢ. 196.—The average height and weight of the public-school children of Boston
    as given by Dr. Bowditch.   For use in public schools these figures should be
    given in place of those in Fig. 195.

CHAPTER XVI.

Report of the Committee on Statistics appointed by the Association in 1885, giving the detailed method of securing measurements, tests, and the condition of the human body.

ANTHROPOMETRIC MEASUREMENTS.

Number.—In order to secure privacy the individual should be entered in the record book by number. As a means of identification the number can be entered in an alphabetical index book opposite the corresponding name, as:

Smith, John H., 526

For further convenience it is advisable to enter the name in a numerical index-book opposite the corresponding number, as:

526, John H. Smith.

Date.—Record the year, month, day and hour, as: Jan., '86, 12, 9 A.M. Where perfect accuracy is desired, note should be made of the time that has elapsed since eating, the occupation of previous hours, and of the temperature of the room.

Age.—Record years and months, as: 21, 9, *i.e.*, twenty-one years and nine months.

Weight.—The weight of the body should be **taken without clothes.** Where **this is** impracticable the weight of the clothes **should be** deducted.

Height.—The height **should** be taken without shoes and with the head uncovered. The head and figure should be held easily erect, and the heels together. This position **is** best secured by bringing the heels, the buttocks, the spine between the shoulders and the back of the head, in contact with the measuring **rod.**

Height of Knee.—The subject should **place** one **foot** on a box or chair of such a height that the knee is bent at a right angle. A box about **12 in.** high is suitable for adults. Press a **ruler upwards with a** force of about one pound against the **hamstring** tendons close to the calf of the leg. **See that the** ruler is held in a position at right **angles to the** vertical rod, and measure the height of **the top of the ruler** from the box.

Height Sitting.—**Let the** subject **sit** on a hard, flat surface about **12** inches high, such as afforded by **a** box or chair, **with the** head and figure easily erect so that the measuring rod will touch the body **at the buttocks,** between the shoulders, and **at** the back **of the** head. Measure the distance from **the box to the vertex.**

Height of Pubes.—With **the** subject standing easily erect on the box or floor, measure up to the lower edge of the pubic bone.

Height of Crotch.—With the subject standing easily erect **on** the **box** or floor facing the vertical rod, press a ruler firmly against the perineum (crotch) and measure the height of the top of the ruler.

Height of Navel.—With the figure and head of the subject erect, measure the height of the center of the cicatrix.

Height of Sternum.—With the figure and head of the subject erect, measure the height of the interclavicular notch.

Girth of Head.—This measurement should be taken around the head with the tape at the upper edge of the eyebrows, over the supra-orbital and occipital prominences. All girths should be made on the skin itself and at right angles to the axis of the body or limb at the point of measurement. No oblique measurements are taken.

Girth of Neck.—With the head of the subject erect, pass the tape around the neck half way between the head and body, or just below the "Adam's apple."

Girth of Chest.—Pass the tape around the chest so that it shall embrace the scapulæ and cover the nipple. The arms of the subject should be held in a horizontal position while the tape is being adjusted and then allowed to hang naturally at the sides. Take the girth here before and after inflation.

Where it is desirable to test the elasticity or extreme mobility of the walls of the chest, a third measurement may be taken after the air has been forced out and the chest contracted to its greatest extent. To test the respiratory power, independent of muscular development, pass the tape around the body below the pectoral line and the inferior angles of the scapulæ, so that the upper edge shall be two inches below the nipples. Take the girth here before and after inflation.

Girth of Waist.—The waist should be measured at the smallest part after a natural expiration.

Girth of Hips.—The subject should stand erect with feet together. Pass the tape around the hips above the pubes over the trochanters and the glutei muscles.

Girth of Thighs.—With the feet of the subject about six inches apart, the muscles set just enough to sustain the equilibrium of the body and the weight distributed equally to each leg in gluteal fold, measure around the thigh just below the nates.

Girth of Knee.—With the knee of the subject straight and the weight of the body equally supported on both legs, measure over the center of the patella.

Girth of Calf.—With the heels down and the weight of the body supported equally on both feet, the tape should be placed around the largest part of the calf.

Girth of Instep.—Measure around the instep at right angles with the top of the foot, passing a point at the bottom of the foot midway between the end of the great toe and back of the heel.

Girth of Upper Arm.—With the arm of subject bent hard at elbow, firmly contracting the biceps and held away from the body in a horizontal position, pass the tape around the greatest prominence. If desirable to find the girth of the upper arm when the biceps is not contracted, the arm should be held in a horizontal position and measured around the most prominent part.

Girth of Elbow.—Taken around the internal condyle of the humerus while the arm of the subject is straight, with the muscles of the forearm relaxed.

Girth of Forearm.—Taken around the largest part. The fist should be firmly clinched and the palm of the hand turned upward.

Girth of Wrist.—With the hands of the subject open and the muscles of the forearm relaxed, measure between the styloid process and the hand.

Breadth of Head.—The breadth of head should be taken at the broadest part. In taking the breadth measurements, stand behind the subject.

Breadth of Neck.—Taken at the narrowest part with the head of the subject erect and the muscles of the neck relaxed.

Breadth of Shoulders.—With the subject standing in a natural position, elbows at the sides, shoulders neither dropped forward nor braced backward, measure the broadest part two inches below the acromion processes.

Breadth of Waist.—Taken at the narrowest part.

Breadth of Hips.—Measure the widest part over the trochanters, while the subject stands with feet together, the weight resting equally on both legs.

Breadth of Nipples.—Taken from center to center with the chest in a natural position.

Depth of Chest.—Taken after a natural inspiration. Place one foot of the calipers on the sternum midway between the nipples, and the other foot on the spine at such a point that the line of measurement is at right angles with the axis of the spinal column. When it is desirable to ascertain the extent of the antero-posterior movement of the chest, measurements may be taken from the same points after the fullest inspiration and after the fullest expiration.

Depth of Abdomen.—Place one foot of the calipers immediately above the navel, the other on the spine at such a point that the line of measurement is at right angles to the axis of the spinal column.

Length of Shoulder to Elbow.—With the arm of the subject bent sharply at the elbow and held at the side, measure from the top of the acromion process to the olecranon. Care should be taken that the measuring rod is parallel with the humerus and not with the external surface of the arm.

Length from Elbow to Finger Tip.—With the arm of the subject bent sharply at the elbow and the rod resting on back of arm and hand, measure from the olecranon process to the tip of the middle finger.

Length of Foot.—Take the extreme length of foot from the end of the first or second toe to the back of the heel, about one inch from the surface upon which the foot rests.

Stretch of Arms.—With the arms of subject stretched out horizontally so that both hands and shoulders are in a line, with one middle finger and the zero end of the measuring rod pressed against the wall, note the point to which the other middle finger tip reaches.

Horizontal Length.—With the heels of the subject pressed hard against a perpendicular wall, with arms at the sides and body resting naturally on a horizontal plane, measure the distance of the apex of the head from the wall.

Capacity of Lungs.—The subject after loosening the clothing about the chest and taking a full inspiration, filling the lungs to their utmost capacity, should blow slowly into the spirometer. Two or three trials may be allowed.

Expiratory Strength.—As before, the subject after loosening the clothing about the chest and filling the lungs completely, should blow with one blast into the manometer. Care should be taken that no air is allowed to escape at the sides of the mouth, and that in expelling the air all the muscles of expiration are brought into play.

Strength of Back.—The subject, standing upon the iron foot-rest with the dynometer so arranged that when grasping the handles with both hands his body will be inclined forward at an angle of 60°, should take a full breath and, without bending the knees, give one hard lift, mostly with the back.

Strength of Legs.—The subject while standing on the foot-rest with body and head erect, and chest thrown forward, should sink down, by bending the knees, until the handle grasped rests against the thighs; then taking a full breath, he should lift hard, principally with the legs, using the hands to hold the handle in place.

Strength of Chest.—The subject with his elbows extended at the sides until the forearms are on the same horizontal plane and holding the dynometer so that the dial will face outward and the indicator point upward, should take a full breath and push vigorously against the handles, allowing the back of the instrument to press on the chest.

Strength of Upper Arms, Triceps.—The subject, while holding the position of rest upon the parallel bars, supporting his weight with arms straight, should let the body down until the chin is level with the bars, and then push it up again until the arms are fully extended. Note the number of times that he can lift himself in this manner.

Strength of Upper Arms, Biceps.—The subject should grasp a horizontal bar or pair of rings and hang with the feet clear from the floor while the arms are extended. **Note the number** of times that he can haul his body up until his chin touches the bar or ring.

Strength of Forearms.—The subject, while holding the dynamometer so that the dial is turned inward, should squeeze the spring as hard as possible, first with the right hand and then with the left. The strength of the muscles between the shoulders may be tested with the same instrument. The subject, while holding the dynamometer on a level with the chest, should grasp it with handles and pull with both arms from the center outward.

Pilosity.—Note the amount of hair on the body and limbs, excluding the head, face and pubes.

Color of Hair.—*Light* (Very Fair, Fair, Light Brown, Brown). *Dark* (Dark Brown, Black Brown, Black). *Red* (Red Brown, Red, Golden).

Color of Eyes.—*Light* (Dark Blue, Blue, Light Blue). *Dark* (Light Brown, Brown, Dark Brown, Black). *Mixed* (Gray, Green).

DIRECTIONS FOR TESTING **THE REFRACTIVE** CONDITION **OF**
THE EYE.

Procure **of any** optician two pairs **of spectacles, one**
with convex glasses, No. + .75 **Dioptric (equal to**
No. +. 48 in the old or English system), and **the other**
with concave glasses, No. + .75 Dioptric. Also obtain
a copy of Monoyer's test letters (a card of **Dr. Den-**
nett's modification of Monoyer's test type may **be pro-**
cured of Meyrowitz Bros. opticians, 295 and 297
Fourth **Ave., New York** City), to be hung **up at 5**
meters **distance, and** a **copy** of Green's astigmatic
lines, in the **form of** a clock **face, to be** hung up at **the**
same distance.

Test :—Seat the subject at **a distance** of five meters
from the test cards, which should be **hung in** a good
light. Examine each eye separately, keeping **the**
other covered by a card **or** small book held in **front**
of, but not touching **it.** Never **press** the **fingers**
against **the closed** lid.

There are ten lines of letters on the test card, **num-**
bered from 1, 2, 3, etc., up to ten 10ths or **1. If now**
the subject can read the **top line, the smallest letters**
on the card, with the right eye (R.E.) alone, his vision
(V.) is recorded as ten 10ths or 1 (V.R.E. **= 1). If he**
sees nothing clearly above the fifth line from the **bot-**
tom, but can read that correctly, then **V.R.E. = .5. If**
he cannot read any **of** the lines, **then V.R.E. = 0.** (*i.e.,*
less than one-10th). **Whatever** the **vision** without
glasses may prove **to be,** *always* *next* put on the *convex*
spectacles and again cover the other eye. **If now he**

can **still** with the right eye see **as** well or better **than** with **no** glasses at all, and can **read** the same line **as** before, he is Hypermetropic (H.) in that eye.   **For example**, if without glasses it **was** found that V.R.E. =. **5**, and now after adding **the** convex glass his V. is improved to .8, the record would be V.R.E. = .5, + H. = .8. But if the vision is neither improved nor made worse by the convex **glass**, the record will **be** thus: V.R.E. = .5, + H. = .5.   **If** the convex glass can be used at all without decreasing the vision, no further testing with this card **is** needed; the subject is **hypermetropic in** that eye.

If it **is** found that the vision **of** the right **eye equals 1 without** glasses, and then the **addition of the** convex glasses blurs the letters, the eye **is** Emmetropic, that is, the vision is normal (V.R.E. = **1**).

If, however, the vision without glasses is less than 1., for instance only .3, and the convex glasses make even that line more indistinct, then put on the *concave* glasses. **If now the** vision is improved so that **a** higher line can be read, for instance the eighth **from** the bottom, the eye is Myopic, or "near sighted," **and** the record will be V.R.E. = .3, + My. = .8. Or again, if the vision without glasses in the left **eye is found** to be .7 and then with the concave glass the top line can be read, the record will stand thus: V.R.E. = .7, + My. = 1. After testing each eye separately, place the record **of one** above the **other**, for example thus:

$$\begin{cases} V.R.E. = 1. \\ V.L.E. = .6, + My. = .9. \end{cases}$$

This completes the testing for simple hypermetropia, myopia and **emmetropia**.

After testing the eyes **as above, if** the vision has not yet been made perfect in either, leave on the proper correcting glass, the convex if there is hypermetropia, or the concave if there is myopia, or use no glass if there is neither; then direct the subject's attention **with** that eye alone, the other being covered, to **the card of** radiating black lines. If he sees one **or more** of the lines running **in** any direction clearer **or** blacker than those at right angles to them, **he** is shown to be astigmatic. Either the perpendicular or the horizontal lines usually **appear** the blacker **to the** astigmatic person. If the previous record **was V.R.E.** $= .7$ and **this** defect is found, then it will **be V.R.E.** $= .7, +$ As. Or if before it read : V.L.E. $= .3, +$ **My.** $= .6$, and astigmatism is found, it will read, V.L.E. $= .3, +$ My. $= .6 +$ **As.** Astigmatism may exist either alone or in **combination with My. or H.** If alone we might **have a** record thus : **V.R.E.** $= .6, +$ **As.** ; V.L.E. $= .4, +$ **As.,** or if with hypermetropia **thus : V.R.E.** $= 7, +$ **H.** $= .7, +$ As. ; V.L.E. $= .6, +$ H. $= .8, +$ As.

To recapitulate, in brief ; **if it is found that V.R.E.** $= 1$, then the R.E. is **either** Emmetropic or Hypermetropic. If emmetropic, the convex glass will markedly impair the vision ; if hypermetropic it will not. If the **V.R.E.** $= .9$ **or** less, then the R.E. is either hypermetropic, myopic, astigmatic, or amblyopic.

1*st*. If **it is H., the convex glass** will **not** greatly impair the vision.

2*d*. If it is My., **the concave glass will improve V.**

3d. If it is As., one of the radiating lines is blackest.

4th. If neither of these defects exists and the V. is less than .7, then Amblyopia or partial blindness may be recorded. It may read thus: V.L.E. $= .6 +$ Am.

Caution.—Always try the *convex* glass. *Never* try the *concave* unless the convex glass blurs the vision.

In the following cases the subject should be recommended to consult an oculist concerning the advisability of wearing glasses : If the vision without any glasses is less than 4 in either or both eyes ; if he complains of weak, watery, or painful eyes, especially in reading, and any degree of hypermetropia or astigmatism is found to exist.

DIRECTIONS FOR TESTING THE COLOR SENSE.

A reliable set of test worsteds of different colors may be procured for $1.25 of N. D. Whitney, 129 Tremont St., Boston. Among these will be found three large test skeins colored light green, purple (pink or rose), and bright red. To make the examination, spread all the worsteds out on a white cloth placed upon a table. First lay the *green* test skein a little to one side of the others, and then tell the subject to throw out of the pile and lay alongside of the test skein all the lighter and darker shades of that color, or all the skeins containing a shade of that color in any degree. Avoid naming the color "green" to him. If he throws out only shades of green or light blues his color sense is normal (C.S.N.) and the test is completed. But if in addition he throws out light grays, or any other shade of gray, or light yellows, salmons, or pinks, he is color-blind. If he handles or fumbles over those shades a good deal and hesitates, as if in doubt about them, but yet does not throw them out, he probably has " feeble color sense" (C.S.F.). The examiner in these cases must use his judgment in making a certain amount of allowance for the stupidity of some persons in understanding what is wanted, especially in the young and uneducated.

If the subject is found to be color-blind, next lay down the purple or rose-colored test skein in place of the green, in order to determine the nature of the defect. Now tell him to throw out all the different shades of that color. If he only throws out pinks and light reds, and shades approaching these, he is only partly color-blind (P.C.B.). But if he throws out decidedly bluish purples, blues, violets, greens, or grays, he is completely color-blind (C.C.B.). Completely red-blind if he throws out the blues, violets, etc.; or green-blind if the grays or greens.

No further testing is needed; but as a matter of curiosity, and to prove the result, the red test skein may next be tried in the same way. If he matches with it browns or greens and grays, he is completely color-blind : dark brown or green if red-blind ; and light brown or green if green-blind.

It is not important to record whether the complete color-blindness is red or green blindness. The following classes may be recorded : Color sense normal = C.S.N.; color sense feeble = C.S.F.; partial color-blindness = P.C.B.; complete color-blindness = C.C.B.

Color-blind individuals should **be** warned against engaging **in** any occupation where **this** defect would prove dangerous or inconvenient.

DIRECTIONS FOR TESTING **THE** CONDITION OF THE EARS.

Use an ordinary watch and a tuning-fork, **letter A or C, as** tests. **Seat the** subject with his right side toward you ; **and** then while the room is perfectly quiet, see how **far off** he can hear the watch tick. Having previously learned by a few experiments what **is** the farthest distance at which the **tick** can be heard **by normal** ears, make that **number of inches the de-**nominator of a fraction, and **the** hearing-distance **of each** person examined thereafter the numerator. Having found the normal distance ($=$ H.D.) to be, for instance, about sixty inches, **and** that of the subject now examined to be, say, **forty** inches, his record for the right **ear** would then be H.D.R.E. $= \frac{40}{60}$. If it had been $\frac{60}{60}$, **or** 1, the ear would be normal. $\frac{80}{60}$ would show an abnormally acute sense of hearing. If the watch could only **be** heard while in *contact* **with his** ear, it would be recorded H.D.R.E. $= \frac{c}{60}$. **If not** heard at all, then H.D.R.E. $= \frac{0}{60}$. Next, test **the** left ear in the same way. Voice sounds in talking will often **be** easily heard by persons quite deaf to the **watch** tick : **so** the latter is **not** always a reliable practical test.

Suppose we have found H.D.R.E. $= \frac{40}{60}$, H.D.L.E. $=$ 1; this implies some deafness in the right ear ; and the tuning-fork will now help us to decide whether the cause lies in some defect of the auditory nerve or internal ear, or in **the** external or middle ear or Eustachian tube. Strike the fork against some solid substance, and then place the end of **the** handle against or between the subject's front **teeth.** If both ears are **normal,** he will probably seem to hear the ringing of the **fork** equally well in both ears. But **if there is a** defect in one ear, he will either seem to hear **it louder** or more feebly in the affected ear. If, as in the case **we** are examining, the fork is heard best in the **deaf** ear, this tells **us** that the deafness is due to **some defect** in the **more** external parts of the organ, and it can probably be corrected by appropriate treatment. **But if** it is heard **best** in the good ear, it goes to prove that the defect in the other ear is more deeply seated and cannot probably be greatly benefited **by** treatment. This effect of the tuning-fork is contrary to what would ordinarily be expected; and it is often **a** matter of surprise **to a** deaf person **to** find that he hears with his teeth apparently better on the deaf side.

We may now add to our record in this case: **T. F. best** R.E. **If it had been** heard equally well **in both ears, we would record: T.F. = N. (or normal).** Where the defect in hearing **is at** all marked, a specialist in ear diseases should be consulted.

Our record in **a** normal case might be thus: **H.D. R.E. = 1, H.D.L.E. = 1, T.F. = N.;** or in an abnormal **case** it might be thus: H.D.R.E. $= 1$, H.D.L.E. $= \frac{0}{60}$, **T.F.** best in R.E. This would imply that the subject was so deaf in the left **ear as not to** be able to hear the watch tick at all, and **the fork** held between the teeth could be heard best in **the good ear; conse-**

quently his trouble is probably **seated** in the deeper structures of the ear, or in the nerve itself, and treat-**ment would** not be expected **to help** him greatly. The tuning-fork need not be tried unless the watch tick shows some defect in hearing.

TO EXAMINE **THE** LUNGS AND HEART.

Procure a Camman's Binaural Stethoscope, Fig. 206. Before the subject tries any of the strength-tests, **let** him be seated, and while the breathing and circulation are easy apply the stethoscope to various parts of the chest. The faint respiratory murmur **heard every-where** will soon become familiar, and any unusual sounds should be noted as abnormalities. These may be crackling, bubbling or whistling sounds of varying intensity. Or the respiratory murmur may be abnor-mally **loud** or entirely absent. Note whether these **sounds change or** disappear with deep breathing after violent exercise.

Next listen to **the** heart sounds. Place the stetho-scope over the apex of the heart, one inch below **and to** the right of the left nipple. Both sounds **should be** heard most distinctly here. Then **place** the in-strument two inches above this spot **and listen.** Then place it two inches below the center of the top of the sternum, or breast-bone, **and** listen in this vicinity. Any abnormal heart sounds **are** apt to be heard most distinctly at one of these points. In organic heart diseases rough grazing or blowing sounds are heard with one or both of the normal heart sounds. Take no notice of **an** arterial murmur heard loudest under the outer half of each collar-bone, which often closely resembles an abnormal heart murmur, especially after violent exercise.

If all the heart sounds are **natural,** then let **the subject take** the arm-tests of pulling up or dipping, and **immediately after** let him be seated again, **and then** listen **to see if the** heart and lung sounds **are still** natural, though intensified by the exertion just **made.** Also note any irregularity in the rhythm of **the heart** sounds or **any intermission** in the beat or **great increase** of rapidity. **There may be such,** as functional disturbances, without **any organic disease.** When the breathing **and heart sounds seem abnormal advise** consulting a physician.

The foregoing rules **for examining the** lungs and heart are taken from the Amherst College Anthropometric Manual, prepared by Dr. Edward Hitchcock, **Director** of the Pratt Gymnasium at Amherst, Mass.

EXAMINATION OF THE LUNGS BY PERCUSSION.

By this method **of examination it is possible to de-**tect certain forms of **disease.**

If the left hand is placed firmly over some part of the thorax and is then struck lightly by the first two **fingers** of the right hand there **is a** resonance that shows whether the lungs are **in a normal or an ab-normal** condition. It requires **practice** to detect **the** various degrees of resonance, **and** this practice the teacher should try to get.

In place of the hands we **should recommend the**

Percussor (see Fig. 197) or rubber-hammer, and the Pleximeter (Fig. 198).

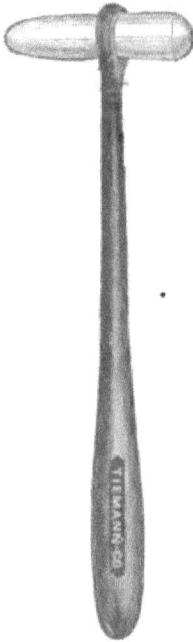

Fɪɢ. 197.
Percussor.

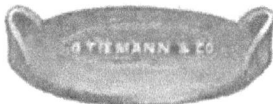

Fɪɢ. 198.
Pleximeter.

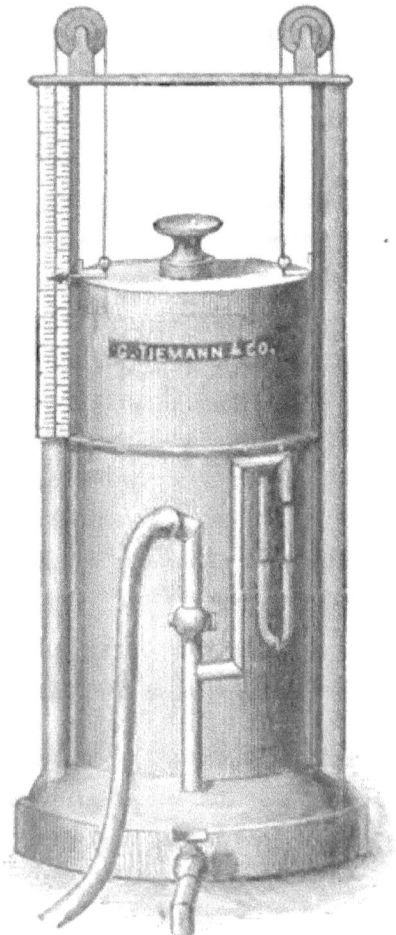

Fɪɢ. 199.
Spirometer.

Fig. 200 represents the chest, back, and leg dyna-mometer.

Fig. 201 represents the hand dynamometer. This

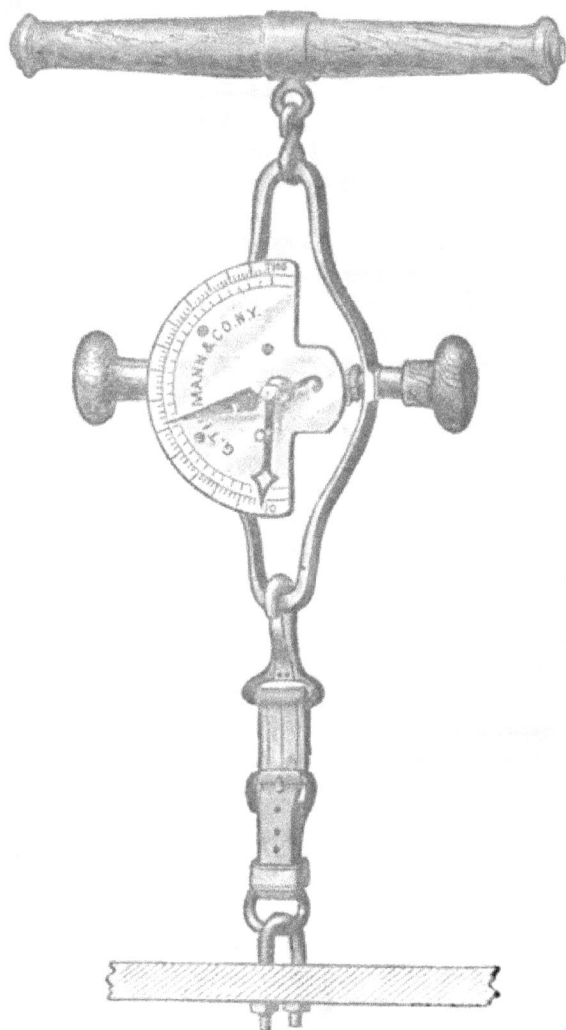

FIG. 200.
Dynamometer for testing the strength of chest, back, and legs.

can also be used as a test for back and legs by attaching handles.

Fig. 202 represents the height-tester. This comes

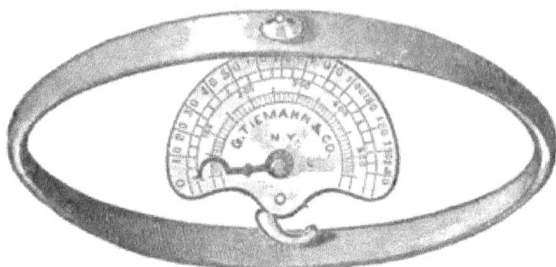

Fig. 201.

Hand dynamometer.

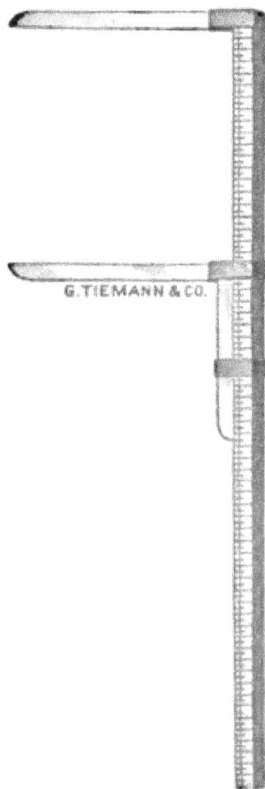

Fig. 203.—Breadth-measure.

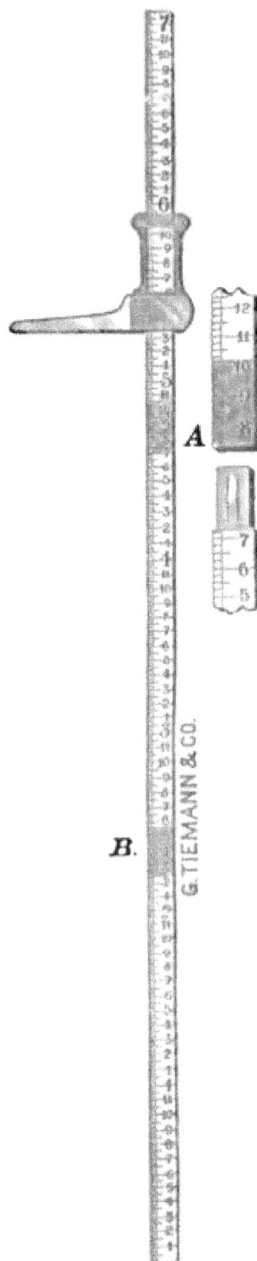

Fig. 202.—Height-tester.

in sections, and is therefore easily carried. The same can be purchased in one piece.

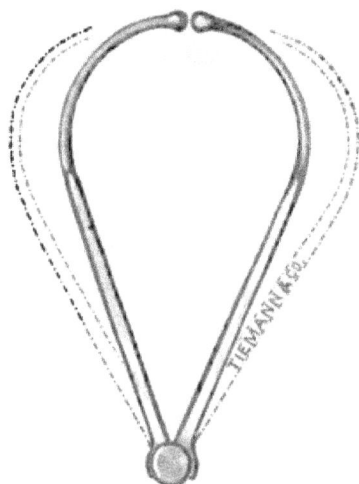

FIG. 204.

Calipers.

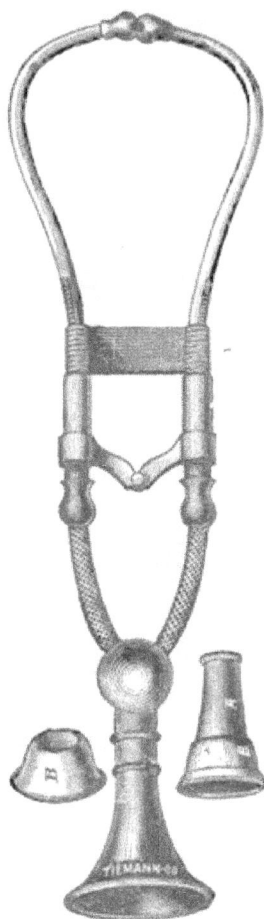

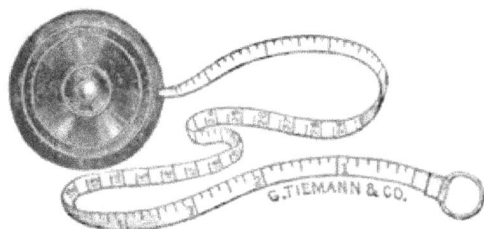

FIG. 205.

FIG. 206.

Fig. 203 represents the breadth-measure.

Fig. 199 shows the Hutchinson's water-spirometer. This is more accurate than the dry machine.

Fig. 204 represents the calipers used in taking diameters of the body.

Fig. 205 represents the tape used in taking measurements.

In Fig. 206 is shown a stethoscope, for examining the lungs and heart.

SPIROMETER.

The spirometer (Fig. 199), which is made upon the same principle as a gasometer, is used mainly to ascertain the capacity of the lungs. It is not possible to tell what the disease of the lungs is, in case a person does not come up to their capacity, nor is the failure on a pupil's part to reach the cubic inches given for his height a sure sign that he has lung trouble. The teacher is safe in saying that any one who reaches or goes above their lung capacity has good lungs.

The use of this instrument requires practice. The greatest respiratory capacity of the lungs is indicated by the amount of air that can be expelled from the lungs at one expiration. This is preceded by a deep inspiration.

It is well to give the pupils several trials on the spirometer before recording their highest blow. A good showing cannot be made if the clothing across the chest is tight, nor can a person make a good record after a hearty meal.

The teacher's attention is called to this fact : that, for every inch in height above four feet, the capacity is increased by eight cubic inches. The author has found that the **lung capacity of females** is not so great as that of males for the same **height; and** while the second table of figures given **is not** authentic, it **is nearer** what females should blow. It may be interesting, in **using** the spirometer, to note the number of respirations in a healthy **person,** and their relation **to the** pulse. **In a** healthy **adult,** the number of respirations ranges from 14 **to 18** a minute. The relation between the pulse and respiration is in the proportion of about 1 to 4 or 1 to 5. This rule, **of course, has** its exceptions.

According to Hutchinson, the principal authority on the use of the spirometer, a **healthy person**

48 inches in height should blow 72 cubic inches.

49	"	"	"	"	80	"	"
50	"	"	"	"	88	"	"
51	"	"	"	"	96	"	"
52	"	"	"	"	104	"	"
53	"	"	"	"	112	"	"
54	"	"	"	"	120	"	"
55	"	"	"	"	128	"	"
56	"	"	"	"	136	"	"
57	"	"	"	"	144	"	"
58	"	"	"	"	152	"	"
59	"	"	"	"	160	"	"
60	"	"	"	"	168	"	"
61	"	"	"	"	176	"	"
62	"	"	"	"	184	"	"
63	"	"	"	"	192	"	"
64	"	"	"	"	201	"	"

65 inches in height should blow 209 cubic inches.

66	"	"	"	"	217	"	"
67	"	"	"	"	225	"	"
68	"	"	"	"	233	"	"
69	"	"	"	"	241	"	"
70	"	"	"	"	249	"	"
71	"	"	"	"	257	"	"
72	"	"	"	"	265	"	"

It has been said, although the author does not vouchsafe for the authority, that Hutchinson gives the following statistics for the lung capacity of females :

A female 48 in. in height should blow 32 cubic in.

"	49	"	"	"	"	40	"	"
"	50	"	"	"	"	48	"	"
"	51	"	"	"	"	56	"	"
"	52	"	"	"	"	64	"	"
"	53	"	"	"	"	72	"	"
"	54	"	"	"	"	80	"	"
"	55	"	"	"	"	88	"	"
"	56	"	"	"	"	96	"	"
"	57	"	"	"	"	104	"	"
"	58	"	"	"	"	112	"	"
"	59	"	"	"	"	120	"	"
"	60	"	"	"	"	128	"	"
"	61	"	"	"	"	136	"	"
"	62	"	"	"	"	144	"	"
"	63	"	"	"	"	152	"	"
"	64	"	"	"	"	160	"	"
"	65	"	"	"	"	168	"	"

A female 66 in. in height should blow 176 cubic in.
    "   67 "   "   "   " 182 "   "
    "   68 "   "   "   " 192 "   "
    "   69 "   "   "   " 200 "   "
    "   70 "   "   "   " 208 "   "

CHAPTER XVII.

A FEW SUGGESTIONS TO TEACHERS.

To be a **successful teacher of** gymnastics, you must believe what you are **teaching.**

You must know the **" hows and** whys" of the subject.

You must know **HOW to teach.**

You should be **well** read on your subject.

You should be fitted physically **for** this work.

A good voice, with **a** knowledge **of how** to use **it, is** essential.

You should have **an** idea of time.

You should be a good disciplinarian.

You should show by your own physique, and the way you handle **it,** that gymnastics will do what you say they will.

You should be an expert in one or more branches of this profession.

If you do not possess the **above** qualifications, you **can** work for them ; and **if** you **work** hard, you will be apt to succeed.

Remember that the science **of** teaching applies to physical as well as mental work ; therefore read the best works on pedagogy.

When teaching, much of your success is due to discipline.

226

Remember **that a rule is good for** nothing unless it is enforced.

You must be determined **to** have **order ;** but there **are two** sides to a question : therefore **do** not be too **hasty** in your decisions.

If you say you will do a thing, do it.

Run your own department. You are worth **more to** your principal **if** you **are not** obliged to **go to him** for **aid in** every little thing.

It is "devoutly **to be** wished" that **any** one who claims **to be a** teacher **of** gymnastics **will** not only present the **subject in** its **true colors, but** that **he** will also teach a correct system.

Gymnastics **may** be taught in **two ways :** one where **the work** is for recreation and fun alone ; the other **where** the exercises are given **to** produce proper **physcial** development ;—the latter being the way **they should be** taught.

As it would be **impossible for a** doctor to prescribe with **safety for a patient without** understanding **the** theory and **practice of** medicine, so it is just **as** impossible for a **teacher to** teach gymnastics **as they** should be taught if she does not understand : **(1) the** location of the various sets of muscles ; **the** names **given to** different parts of the physique, **such** as front upper arm, upper back, and waist ; the result of over-development **opment of particular** sets **of** muscles, and the most common **physical defects caused** by this over-development ment ;—and **(2) what** exercises should be given to **remedy these defects.**

The exercises given in this **book,** with the method of teaching them, are based upon this knowledge. All technical terms are avoided. The body is so divided (and these divisions are named) that children will readily understand them.

The rules for developing any particular portion of the muscular system can be easily comprehended. They are described so that a teacher can easily enforce them by appealing to the simple reasoning power of children. The few common defects mentioned will be noticed by teachers any day if their attention is called to them.

They can be overcome if teachers will do their part, and if the parents will assist ; but teachers can not do the work alone.

The teacher's opinion influences children in this respect much more than is supposed ; so that "Train up a child as it should go" is as applicable here as elsewhere.

Moreover, a child will adhere to a wrong opinion if it thinks it is right; thus, it is necessary that the teacher should understand this work, and teach it correctly.

The success of physical training depends, not so much on the parents of to-day, because it is new to them, but on the coming fathers and mothers, because they have had the experience and appreciate its value. Again, if this subject is presented as it should be, the most conservative will admit that "There is something in it."

Teachers are needed who can do this.

When parents come to consider that there are over

20,000 students in our medical colleges, and that these embryo doctors are to treat the aches and pains that in many cases could have been prevented by obeying the laws of physical education ; when they think that a fraction of the large sums paid to physicians to cure disease would have given their children preventive gymnastic training ;—we may look for stronger support in that direction.

On the other hand, there must be a decided change in our methods of teaching gymnastics : we must appeal to the sense, and not to the vision. The teacher who drills a class entirely for show will not long be successful. She must offer something that is thoroughly-practical. If the teacher allows her pupils to think for one minute that they are drilled in these exercises for the novelty, her work must sooner or later become unpopular. A pupil is not permitted to think that arithmetic is taught for the fun of the thing ; nor should he be allowed to think that gymnastics are so taught.

One of the strongest arguments that we can present is the effect that exercise has upon the nervous system and brain. There is an intimate relation between the mind and body.

We know that exercise develops the muscles ; and through the muscular system, training affects the growth of nerves.

We have grounds for believing that by this means we can develop the brain substance itself, and thus put it in better condition for its mental education.

A clumsy, awkward boy who is mentally sluggish

can be so **quickened** by gymnastic drill **that he will** eventually **succeed** in intellectual work and **excel in** athletics too.

COSTUME.

When pupils **exercise daily, the** time being limited, **and** pass from **the class-room to** the gymasium, no time can be spared **for a change in** costume. **Nor, in-** deed, is it **absolutely** necessary **that a change be made.** The exercises **given in this** book can be taken **by pupils in** their **street dress. The** author drills six or **seven** hundred pupils **daily in light gymnastics,** yet **wears no** special **suit.**

Up to a certain age, girls can exercise in **their school dress with** ease.

It is not until the **corset makes** its appearance, and **the** waist **is** made tighter, that there is restriction **of movement;** and then it **is generally** noticed when **an** attempt **is** made **to raise the arms above** the head. The same **trouble is not noticed in** boys when exer- cising, as **they fortunately** do **not wear** the yoke **of** fashion.

Teachers can, **to some** extent, **modify the dress** worn by girls. **They can** persuade them **to have** changes made that will permit them **to at** least raise **the arms** above the **head.** They **can prove** that cer- tain dress-waists **give** form and figure, **as** well as cor- sets do. The corset can not be abolished—it **has** come **to stay;** but it can be modified.

It is of course better that pupils don **a** regular cos- **tume, if** the opportunity is given.

For mixed classes, boys can **wear a** sailor or tennis

shirt, knickerbockers, and rubber-soled shoes. Flannel pants that buckle at the ankle and are held up by a belt are sometimes preferred, as long stockings are not then required.

Girls should wear a costume of three pieces— loose waist, skirt, and trousers of some flannel. The trimming may be put on the suit as desired. It is better that suits be alike, and that the ends of the skirts be the same distance from the floor.

The rubber-soled shoe has been condemned on the ground that it heats the foot. So it does, but it does no harm. Exercise heats the body, too. We can not draw the line at the feet. Rubber-soled shoes are safer.

When the sexes work by themselves, boys should wear close-fitting garments of some pliable material. Cotton or worsted tights answer the purpose. Girls and young ladies should wear the divided skirt, especially if they are to do any heavy work or exercise on the bars, rings, etc.

Several styles of costumes are shown in the Manual.

CHAPTER XVIII.

MUSIC.

FROM the beginning of time, people have loved music: they have been able to throw more life into their work if inspired by its exhilarating strains. **In** dancing, every movement is animated; **in** marching, a step becomes lighter **and more elastic if** accompanied **by** music. In fact, melody **kindles the** enthusiasm and adds new energy to motion.

Dancing without music is dead; yet dancing is one form of gymnastic exercise. Much **of** its popularity is due **to the** harmony that follows it. All light gymnastic exercises **should be,** where practicable, executed **to** music. **The advantage** of such accompaniment will **be** apparent after **its** successful adoption.

We wish to say but **a** few words to the teacher **regarding** this part of the work:

If you are to choose between **poor music** and no music, choose the latter.

Engage a musician who **is not** entirely confined to **notes.**

The pianist must be able to watch the instructor.

Never meet a class for exercise until your accompanist has **had an** opportunity to practice with you beforehand. **You** must know your player; while he, in turn, must clearly **understand** your signals and commands.

Remember that playing **for** gymnastics **is a profession.** It must be well learned. Therefore, use patience with the **one** who thus assists you **if he is a** beginner.

Every command must be heard by the accompanist as well as by the class.

To the Accompanist.—You must excel in TIME. You must watch the gymnasium teacher, and not your notes.

You should have a variety of pieces.

Do not play classical music for gymnastics.

You should understand the order of exercises.

Use a little care in the selection of your music. Choose that which is inspiring.

Learn to accent certain notes.

Be able to change easily, and without effort, from quick to slow time. You can easily change a polka or galop to march time.

You fill a difficult and important position : do not think otherwise. You need a powerful touch.

These suggestions may sound somewhat arbitrary, but they are based on unpleasant experience ; they are not ideal.

Teachers will be saved much embarrassment if they will only heed them.

Polkas, galops, and waltzes are easier to get than good marches. The author has named a few that will be found to contain the requisite "snap." Nos. 3, 4, and 5 are used for runs :

1. Grand Festal March. A. J. Powell.

2. Boulanger March.   A. H. Rosewig.
3. Patrol Comique.   T. Hendley.
4. Secret Love.
5. Little Pickaninny or Helloh Babby.
6. Dancing in the Barn.
7. Anvil Chorus.   " Il Trovatore."
8. Ivanhoe Commandery March.   C. D. Blake.
9. Adelphi March.   A. S. Lewis.
10. Northern Route March.   C. C. Smith.
11. Marche du Nuit.   Gottschalk.
12. Spirit of the Age.   A. E. Warren.
13. Travesty March.   J. C. Minton.
14. Marche des Tambours.   S. Smith.
15. Criterion March.   C. H. Marcy.
16. Aphrodite Schottische.   A. N. La Brie.
17. Mandolin Polka.
18. Brooklyn Bridge, or Nineteenth-century Wonder.
19. Drum Taps.
20. Evangeline.   Geo. Schleifforths.

LIBRARY OF THE UNIVERSITY OF CALIFORNIA

168447

www.ingramcontent.com/pod-product-compliance
Lightning Source LLC
Chambersburg PA
CBHW030313270326
41926CB00010B/1352